Rose-Tinted – M.y S.tory

"The problem with you is you see everything through rose-tinted glasses.

The rest of the world must deal with reality."

Kezia Kecibas

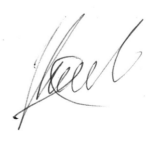

ISBN: 978-1-7398834-0-9

Produced by **samanthahoughton.co.uk**

Disclaimer

To protect the identities of parties that do not wish to be named or identified; names and locations have been changed by the author.

This book contains general information about the treatment of MS based on the experience of the author. It is not meant as medical advice, diagnosis or treatment, and you must not rely on the information in this book as an alternative or substitute to medical advice from your doctor or other professional healthcare provider. If you have any concerns or questions regarding your health or that of your children or adults within your care, you should seek advice from your doctor.

If you think you may be suffering from any medical condition, you should seek immediate attention from your doctor or other professional healthcare provider. You should never delay seeking medical advice, disregard medical advice or discontinue medical treatment based on information in this book.

To the extent that you rely on any information in this book, you assume all risks involved in such reliance.

Table of Contents

Foreword

My Story is exactly that. This book has been written from my perspective of life and how I remember past events. Under no circumstance should any statistics or medical information stated be taken as absolute. I am most definitely not a scientist or expert of any kind. I have mainly blagged my way through life so far.

Where I am not judgemental in any way, shape or form, there will always be someone that may be offended. If this is the case, lighten up!

Where I try hard to avoid it, the odd obscenity may creep into my written word. This is and always will be, expressive and by no means a lack of articulation.

Please simply see it as: my thoughts, my words, my writing, My Story.

Acknowledgements

This book is a direct result of events and experiences that would not have happened without the advice and support of so many friends, family and kind-hearted strangers, not to mention the Doctors and staff of the A.A. Maximov Department of Hematology and Cellular Therapy.

So many have helped keep my life Rose-Tinted, if I were to include every one of you, I would definitely need more than one book. For now, I hope the universe throws many karma points your way.

In particular, I would like to thank the following charitable organisations:

AIMS (Auto Immune and Multiple Sclerosis)

Leicestershire MS Therapy Centre

The Oddfellows

MS Society

MS Research Treatment and Education

Dedication

For Liz, our third Musketeer.

Author Bio

Kezia was born and grew up in Cambridge. Since learning to write, she was often found with a pen and paper in hand, declaring her intent to be a writer. Archaeology was not in her vocabulary at this point and digging was not deemed lady like. She moved to study at De Montfort University and graduated with a BA(hons) in Contemporary Theatre. She had always been an active sportswoman until she was diagnosed with MS at the age of 25. Since then, she has taught Positive Thinking and Mental Well-being alongside running her Holistic Therapies business.

During a routine Neurology consultation, she received the negative prognosis that within a couple of years she would inevitably be using a wheelchair. The literal translation of her surname Kecibas (from Turkish) is Goat head, meaning stubborn. Being told what is inevitable, would always be like a flame to blue touch paper for Kezia. In 2019, she underwent Stem Cell Treatment in Moscow to arrest the typical chronic progression of the disease. Being a big believer in karma points, the hope of potential improvements was always on the cards. With her usual rose-tinted outlook on life, she wouldn't just stop the MS - she'd literally be running off the plane that she landed back to the UK on.

Praise For...

Kezia's book is an honest and open account of her journey with MS and HSCT. Her writing portrays bravery and shows strength of character. **Katrina Morley**

I can honestly say that was a fabulous and truthful account of your ms life and your struggle. Straight from the heart and telling it truly just how it should be. I honestly admire your strength, courage and your bravery - you never gave up even though I'm sure you wanted to at times. Your two not so little people kept you battling on, and as you said, "I'm doing this as their mum for them." I applaud you, my beautiful Kezia, your book was beautiful to read, and I feel so honoured. I've laughed, but I also cried in my mind because I know how you have fought. After all, you are one hell of a lady. Be super proud of yourself because you are one of life's beautiful inspirational people, and I love you.

When you came to the ward, I knew you were someone who would not give up and be in a wheelchair. I remember you saying that you need your legs to work for your kids, and by god, you have bloody shown them all and also, you have done it for you. You've shown those suffering from this disease that there is hope out there if you get off your arse and find it as you did. **Gail Dexter Mcewan, Outpatient Ward Coordinator**

Not knowing much about MS, this book opened my eyes to the toll this illness took on Kezia's physical and emotional health. As a reader, I felt honoured that Kezia had taken off her rose-tinted glasses and let me into her struggles. The clear images I had of the treatment centre in Russia was made possible through the vivid descriptions in the book. Kezia's words made it come to life. Wow, what a read and thank you for letting me into your world! **Sarah Jones, Mental Health Nurse**

Fascinating, gripping and emotive, I couldn't put this book down! It tells how MS progresses and the amazing progress being made regarding treatment. It makes you question your attitude toward disability while highlighting the significant link between mental health and physical well-being. I think we could all do with a 'f**k it bucket' in life and stop letting inner fears prevent us from striving for what we want to achieve.

Gripping! This book gives insight into the world of MS and disability as a whole. Very thought-provoking, with lots of poignant messages that would serve us all well in life to take on board.

Touching and brilliant. This book so eloquently sums up a topic that can easily be avoided... Disability! Adding a humorous slant to living with MS brings it home what daily challenges are faced, but how the right outlook in life can mean you are still able to achieve your life goals if you focus and find your ways of adapting to the challenges life throws at you. **Liz Hall**

1

The Signs

My legs had just decided that they'd had enough, so I sat on the low-level wall outside the bright fluorescent garage that I had spotted about three strides previously. Luckily it wasn't raining. I was on my way back from the gym, which was not an irregular thing. I'd done the usual; the bike, rowing machine, treadmill and weights. I was on the walk back to my current abode, an over-priced three bed, which had been altered with minimum effort to accommodate five students and moreover, five students' monthly rent. I wonder if perhaps the body had an auto-function to avoid humiliation. To collapse here, on this road, buzzing with students attracted to the many bars offering cheap multi-coloured shots and BOGOF alcopops would be awful. It really should not have been a concern for a third-year drama student. Perhaps if I had poured cheap cider over myself, people would have just hurdled over my body. Fortunately, all of this just occurred in my over-creative theatrical brain. The mundane reality was that I just sat on the wall outside the garage. As I conjured up reasons for my dead legs and contemplated how long this may last, I pretended to look at my phone and I rang one of my equally ripped off house mates.

"Come join me, I'm just sat on the wall and my legs won't work. I've just been to the gym; think I must have over done it."

My flatmate, the very eccentric and fabulous Mr Rios came rushing over from the house. "Umm Kezia, what are you doing? Just come home," he quipped in his strong Spanish accent. Then followed with a slight interjection of laughter "You did too much at the gym?"

"Just come and sit with me" I replied, trying to mask my steadily increasing frustration. We sat and chatted. Eventually my legs woke up and we headed back towards Lavender Road. If the name of the house matched to its standards, Nettle Ditch really would have been more fitting. The five of us had tried our best to make it homely. A cheap eighties sunset poster, had been sello-taped over our backdoor. I had purchased a floral padded toilet seat for the downstairs loo which was tucked away in the damp, cold, downstairs garage, almost as if it were hiding in shame.

My legs turning numb was not the first time this sort of thing had happened and this incident took me back to an old memory. For a module of my Contemporary Theatre degree we did a twelve hour vigilant. Twelve hours of continual movement, possibly to see the body's response. I do question whether this was a student welfare tick box health exercise rather than a well thought out cultural module. I am by no means complaining, I love the bizarre. The quirkiness of the university professors is what made me chose DMU over a well-established London University with West End links. The following day and for several weeks after this event, my legs suffered with shooting pains that ran the length of and up both sides - I headed to the doctors. "Probably shin splints - just rest," he declared nodding.

It seemed like a fair diagnosis.

Resting was not something that came naturally

to me. When I wasn't sat in a lecture hall with green-faced hungover students, or at a rehearsal with half of the cast in a similar state - the other half in super keen and eager mode - I was at the gym. I worked out mostly solo but I occasionally went along with my flamboyant flatmate Mr Rios. The gym was my time to think about nothing. I whacked on some shorts and turned the music volume up high before stepping onto the treadmill. Looking around the gym, a lot of the girls seemed to be plastered in makeup. It was quite clear that this was a place to not only drop a few pounds, but to also pull someone. To be fair, it was more than possible their appearances were remnants from a lairy all-nighter.

At school, I'd also been fairly active and had mixed groups of friends. The three popular girls and I got on really well but I didn't want to be part of that clique. I had my geeky friends, my sporty best mate and my (a long time ago in Cambridge) ethnic minority friends too. I was confident and well liked, so I was a rare child that didn't get bullied. The odd comment about tree trunk legs was quickly crushed by any one of my friendship groups.

Being half Turkish meant my body hair was dark so more noticeable but it also meant I had a huge dark curly mass on my head that looked fab with little to no effort. Back at home, I remember standing in my green and white crop top set, on the black and white tiled vinyl bathroom floor facing the bath. The wall above was decorated by my own fair hands using a felt tip blower and a multitude of sea stencils and colours. My favourite was the blue octopus, tentacles spread to meet teeny orange fish and yellow star fish. Mum came in smiling with some tubes of hair removal cream. I just stared at her. She had studied Biology, she must surely know about Darwin; the hair was still there for a reason! She smothered both of my legs in freezing cold cream and it absolutely stank. Why would people do this to themselves? I stood there cold, covered in stinky cream in my new crop top set (for some reason to wear under my t-shirt), very uncomfortable, even if this was for only about five minutes. Well, if this was what made her happy who was I to argue? Mum then took a flannel and soaked it under the tap and wiped off the putrid smelling cream along with my leg hair.

At school the next day, my year group were standing huddled on the sports field. I, in my moss green netball skirt, matching knee-high socks - but minus my warming leg hair.

Did no-one know about Darwin?? Hello…

I never got anxious about being picked last, I am almost positive that many of my peers would grow up to be adults with anxiety due to being the last one picked at every P.E. lesson.

I was never chosen for the 100 metres; although I was now a lot lighter and streamlined thanks to my Mum's cream antics, I was by nature, curvy and short. Mum always kept assuring me I would be tall - my feet were huge after all. We had attempted Clarks several times but she soon discovered it was best to go with a ladies Italian style shoe. Italians must have larger feet she would say. Regardless of this, I knew I'd be shooting up during my next growth spurt.

It wasn't long before I was whisked away by my sporty bestie calling my name. I stepped away from the huge mass of anxious students and over to the side of the chosen. I was continually selected for the long-distance runs and relay team as well as right wing for hockey and netball. I tried to avoid basketball at all costs, football too but another one of my best friends was super sporty and would beg me to join in, so occasionally I'd succumb.

In addition to the above I was a member of the boys' volleyball team but for legal reasons, in competition, we had to be a mixed volleyball team (even though I was the only girl). I also loved trampolining. The principle's daughter and I teamed up and performed a synchronised sequence in competitions. We were far from Olympic standard athletes but we always got through to the final four teams.

Then there was another "leg numbing" incident.

It was the summer break from Uni and I'd headed back down south to stay with my mum. She had moved away from our three bedroomed council house in the middle of Cambridge to live with my stepdad in the countryside. It offered quieter and cheaper living but was void of life as far as my student eyes could perceive. My mum had just managed to land herself a job running a new nursery school, also in the middle of nowhere, it was opening day. The multi-coloured nursery walls were dry and the teeny bean bags were placed next to an array of multi-national dolls and books with different cultural relevance.

Mum had run her own Montessori school before the days that I came along, so she was in her element. The open day was to attract young families, who in turn, would be paying out cash for my mum and her team to watch their little blessings whilst they went to work – all so they could afford to pay for such an honour. The weather had been kind and the little darlings, accompanied by their soon to be financially burdened parents had been suitably charmed. As an extra feature they'd hired a trampoline. I had been very restrained for the whole day. I smiled politely and promoted the merits of my Mum's abilities with children, re-visiting my childhood stories for the reassurance of the parents - my work was done.

With only an hour or so left, I looked over at the trampoline before heading towards it and climbing on excitedly. I spent about an hour effortlessly doing all the tricks and manoeuvres I'd learnt. Having performed a front drop, straddle, tuck and half twist, I then came to a sudden stop. As my feet touched the centre of trampoline, I felt an excruciating pain and crumpled onto the trampoline. As my breathing deepened, my eyes filled with tears. I lay flat out on the trampoline and wondered what I could possibly have done. I didn't understand. The tears kept falling as the pain increased - I found myself surrounded by some concerned parents and a few were ushering their children away. There was no blood, but the sight of me quietly sobbing in the centre of a trampoline during the nursery opening day must have been quite an unexpected sight. I'm not sure if I passed out from the pain but I was pretty much carried to the car. Squished into the front seat of my stepdad's blue Fiat Panda we raced towards civilisation. This was another reason people should live in towns. We seemed to hit every single bump upon every meander on every turn of the roads. The English countryside clearly seems to not have any that are straight and flat. Where were these magnificent Roman roads when you needed them?

Later, I found out that my kneecap had slid out of place and sliced across my anti-cruciate ligament. It was unbelievably painful but on the "Kezia Pain Scale" not the worst pain I've felt to date; at the time however it was a tad sore. The doctors removed the shredded tissue and various other squidgy pieces. I had to learn to walk for the second time, firstly when I was a toddler and then after this unwanted hindrance.

One year later, my friend Sam and I regularly went out dancing in night clubs. Sam was outgoing and I was a drama student - we liked attention. We had always marvelled at the running jump in Dirty Dancing when Baby runs, is lifted into the air and into the most amazing, graceful pose. We decided this was a great idea, Sam was robust, so we tried it out every time we went out. It was amazing - we were amazing! We used to clear the dance floor. I would smile sweetly and just politely ask people to step to one side. It was quite incredible how agreeable people were. Sam would stand at one side of the, politely emptied, dance floor and I would run all the way across, leap into the air and she would catch me in the most fabulous of poses. We did this on every night out. It was our thing.

My young mum and stepdad came to stay for the weekend, along with a delightfully silly family friend who I like to refer to as the Buddhist with ice cream. A cleverly ironic nickname as he is a Buddhist and gave me ice cream. Sam and I thought it would be fun to take our slightly older gang clubbing. We all entered the dark night club with its sticky floor, possibly earlier than usual so it wasn't difficult to find a clear running space. Sam and I went to do our usual trick, when my stepdad said "I'll catch you."

Famous last words. I lined up, I ran and I leapt into the air but there was not the usual welcome from my Mr Swayze. I fell onto the claggy club floor with an almighty thud. My knee went again. The bouncer, possibly recognising me as I was a regular, got me a chair, which I sat on for a while before being driven off to A&E by Patrick fucking Swayze. As I squeezed into the front seat of a now upgraded (slightly larger) Fiat Punto and raced to the hospital on nice non-bumpy "Roman" roads -

again, holding my knee as tears soaked my face. Unsurprisingly, I managed to damage my knee quite badly again. I hadn't broken it but apparently it would have been better if I had. My knee had been holding itself together and now it wasn't - Deja vous. The incredible surgeon managed to take some hamstrings (presumably my own) and replace the anti-cruciate ligament. I was told strictly no skiing, I could live with that.

2

An Unexpected Surprise

My university days came to an end as quickly as they'd started. I had lived on a diet of Bacardi and noodles but I'd been physically active and drank water whenever I was at the gym, so figured that made up for it. Like most, I look back with a smile and a sadness that it's all over. I had graduated in Contemporary Theatre with a 2.1 BA Honours degree. In the eyes of society, I was a grown-up which meant I should get a proper job using all the skills I'd learnt.

I say this with a huge smirk on my face. I had certainly grown more confident. After all, only a blossoming theatre student would climb into the water fountain in the centre of the town hall square, persuading passers-by to write their wishes on scraps of paper, before then tying them with ribbons to the surrounding trees. By this I refer to the paper not the people. That said, it might well have bumped that module up to an A star. Perhaps my dissertation would put me in good stead with a future employer? Unsurprisingly, I had to go to the most "far out" of our lecturers to support my dissertation, "Gender role reversal - a comparison between Shakespearean theatre and Kabuki." I wasn't ready to grow-up, just yet. A fellow thespian-graduate and I, decided we would go travelling together. A cliché plan for those still unwilling to start a proper career. I was excited and I felt the adrenalin pumping. I just had to earn a bit of cash for the flight to wherever.

I sat on the worn out, second hand, 3-seater sofa of my slightly less-overpriced property. After all, I had the knowledge and experience of a graduate. It was Wednesday, which meant it was job's day in the local paper. As I flicked through I could smell the inky scent of a freshly printed newspaper. Usually this smell would be accompanied with vinegar and chips; not today though, I was on a mission. I sieved through many adverts - I needed big money fast. "Ah ha sales, of course." This one read "immediate start, set pay with chances of bonuses." It sounded good to me.

I rang and arranged an interview. It was only a five-minute walk from my current abode. I'd dressed in loose fitting black trousers and black strap-on flats. My days of wearing Spice-girl shoes or even tiny heels were over. My poor knees had gone through enough and I did not fancy crutches again. I recalled my post trampoline physio session – it had been like something from a horror film. The physio, a petite blonde, who I knew secretly wore ten-inch heels when she was out, offered me a trampette. This was a teeny trampoline used to strengthen your leg muscles, as opposed to filling you with fear and causing post-traumatic stress.

My hair was tied up neatly into a ponytail. The dark mass of curls looked like they might try and escape any minute but for now they were tidy. I made my way up the five concrete steps and noticed the board ahead stating which floor belonged to whom. I stepped into the lift and pressed button number six to the top floor. Ping. I stepped out and was greeted by a huddle of girls of varying ages all giggling and laughing. The scent of quality perfume and cigarettes followed them as they stepped into the lift I'd just abandoned.

A smart looking chap stood up from his chair

and smiled. He wore a pin-striped suit, with an accompanying black t-shirt underneath. Deja vous thoughts of being stood in the bathroom in my crop top wondering why I had to wear it under my top, flooded my mind. His aroma was much more pleasant than the cream I'd been soaked in I can assure you.

"Head that way, you're looking for Sarah."

I did as I was told. There were many desks and many people all yabbering away. Each table was stacked up with piles of open magazines and papers. This didn't look overly-promising, were they all wanting another job already I wondered?

There was an office at the end of the corridor of loud women and I knocked on the glass panelled door. A tall slim lady in a black suit, with flowing jet black waist length straight hair opened the door to allow me in. "Hi, I'm Sarah, take a seat" she gestured. Her makeup was flawless and she was obviously a gym bunny. She didn't look as if she would have to make any effort to pull someone at the gym, or anywhere for that matter. She had clearly just stepped out of a magazine, rather like the ones I'd just passed by. I wasn't nervous at all.

Theatrical auditions served to harden you up to take knock backs. To be fair I hadn't had many. She quizzed me about my interests. I replied in standard mundane interview spiel - I enjoyed reading and socialising. When asked my biggest flaw, I explained that I was too competitive. It was a smasher of an answer for a sales job. She stood up from her desk and put out her hand - I started in the morning.

I got to work early, remembering which direction to take from the interview. As I walked with purpose towards the office door, a smiley lady stopped me, "You're working with me."

She handed me a piece of paper with a block of written text and beckoned me to sit. I was given a phone and a stack of magazines. It didn't take me long to learn what was the script and by the end of the day I knew it by heart - I was an actress after all. I was selling advertising space. I was used to people and phone calls didn't faze me so it wasn't long before I was taking card details from the customers at the other end of the line. Actors adapt to their roles for shows, I just adapted myself to this scenario. I was an unusually liked cold caller and the sales came thick and fast.

It wasn't long before I realised retention rates were low for most of the team; those that didn't hit their targets were only just making minimum wage. I didn't struggle; my weekly sales target went quickly from selling £500 to £1000 then to £2500. Considering customers could purchase an advert for £50 - I was on fire. Sarah liked me, in fact, I would go as far as to say that she loved me. I was earning her a lot of money after all.

It was a Monday morning and I flicked through pages of the magazines, staring at the adverts looking for inspiration to decide on my feature for the week. I decided on the cottages and staycations section. As I looked down at the pages, the words and images kept blurring, I couldn't focus. I'd never really had any problems with my eyes - I wore reading glasses but that was it. I hadn't had any headaches either so I didn't understand. Perhaps I was not sleeping enough? I'd hardly been out drinking though. Maybe it was just too many late nights? I could cut out the caffeine and replace my regular tea with a herbal variety, ugh – that was not remotely tempting. It was probably best to get an eye test I said to myself. I went over to Sarah's office to see if she would let me out earlier that day to go to the opticians. I felt genuinely worried and she must have seen the concern on my face and agreed. I made the call straight away and managed to get an appointment later that day.

The receptionist was lovely - I wouldn't have been surprised if having heard my shaky voice on the phone was why she'd offered me an appointment so quickly. I left the opticians with advice to check the monitor on my computer as my prescription hadn't changed. I was to return if it happened again.

The next day Sarah marched into the office with some new recruits. It was halfway through the week and none of the current team were doing well and half of them hadn't sold anything. I was close to hitting two grand already. What can I say? People liked me.

"Everyone listen to Kezia," she ordered in her sharp cut-throat voice, "she's already close to target."

Targets meant bonuses and bonuses equalled an air fare. This was a mantra I repeated to myself daily.

In front of my audience in the office, I picked up the phone and scrolled to the back of the Countryfile magazine. As I glanced through the adverts, I spotted a lovely Labrador painting. I typed the number of the talented artist into the phone and I was away;

"Hi my name is Kezia and I work for the Echo. I love your work - do you always work with watercolour?"

This was generally how it would go, obviously it

wasn't necessarily dog paintings but you get the gist.

People interested me and hearing my genuinely inquisitive voice they chatted and they bought. Within six months I was promoted and was given my own paper. The new role also came with its own petrified workforce of four. I gave them the standard script but taught them my way. I was earning good money, all my bonuses and a bit extra whenever one of my team hit their targets. It allowed me to save for travelling and still be able to party hard on Friday and Saturday nights.

Monday morning, as always, came round quickly. Back in the office, one of the girls working for me appeared extra nervous. She was really struggling with sales. I pulled her to one side "What's on your mind? What are you worried about?"

"I think I'm pregnant," she replied looking teary.

I smiled "Okay, at lunchtime go to the Pound Shop and buy yourself a pregnancy test, I think because your stressing your body's gone on strike." I've no idea how I knew about stress and cycles.

"Come back, do the test, it will say negative and then you can just crack on with your day and earn some bloody money," I laughed.

She just looked at me nervously, "you'll tell everyone."

"Why would I?" I replied trying to reassure her. "Okay, go and get two tests. I'll take one and you take one. I'm the manager," I boomed in a dramatic over-the-top manner (with accompanied grandiose arm gestures) "I'm not allowed to be taking pregnancy tests." I said with a smile.

Off she tottered at lunchtime and came back with two pregnancy tests and true to my word, we both headed for the ladies. She did a test and I did one too. She shouted through the cubicle door, sounding relieved "Phew, you're right, I'm not."

I looked down at the test I was holding, still sat on the porcelain throne. Two lines, positive; surely not? I felt sick, this couldn't be right surely. I was not ready to be a grown up. Kids meant you had to be a grown up. I was in my early twenties, I was going travelling - the test must be wrong. After a rather distracted afternoon at work, I took another test that I picked up from a little shop on the way home. It said negative and I was relieved - I couldn't be a mum, I was still a kid myself.

After university, a guy I'd met there who I got on really well with and I, were two of the remaining few without a place to live so we'd got an overpriced place together. He made me belly laugh like no one else and he liked pub quizzes and clubbing too. We thought we'd just see if we could make a go of it, just until I went travelling. Motherhood and Sambuca shots were not compatible. Anyway, I had plans to party hard, then foster when I turned thirty. Anyhow, there were already plenty of little people in the world. Plus, I'd seen the Battersea dogs home advert - in fact, it was in my paper last week. Dogs weren't just for Christmas - I presumed the same applied for kids too.

I waited until my housemate / new fella got in and I shoved one of the pillows from the couch up my top. "What do you reckon?" I joked and told him of the many tests, reassuring him and myself that I wasn't pregnant. He persuaded me to do another test that night. That one came back undetermined.

"Perhaps go to a clinic?" he suggested.

I really did not need this. I rang the number I'd just found in the phone book that was routinely placed on my doorstep. I got a taxi as I had no idea where this "clinic of doom" was.

I sat in the waiting room with a handful of nervous others, also trying not to catch anyone else's eye. My name was called, I shuffled into the tired looking clinical room. The walls looked like a pale yellow but it may have just been dirt. I handed the nurse my teeny pot of wee I'd produced on demand and she disappeared off with it. She returned after what felt like a decade, with a poker face. "The hormone level is so low that I think you were pregnant, but it was in its early stages and you've lost it."

I didn't know how I felt about this. I wasn't expecting to have a baby - I had too many countries to visit and too many nights out to be had. My relationship had only just started after all but part of me felt sad; something I wasn't expecting. I took a deep breath in and gulped. I smiled politely and left the clinic. As neither of us had planned to have children this early in our lives, this became an unspoken occurrence so avoided any awkward discussions.

Work carried on, I hit my weekly targets but I started having more chilled out weekends. However, I had noticed the tops of my legs often felt numb, so I made an appointment at the doctors. Tuesday, the day of my appointment, arrived. I went to work as normal. As I walked into the office I sensed a horrid atmosphere. Some of the "sister" papers hadn't been selling well and the new recruits had not yet mastered their sales techniques. Our weekly pep talk began. Sarah called out a girl's name and proceeded to screech about targets and bonuses. I stood up "I quit."

I didn't know where the words came from. Sarah's face softened, "Kezia, you're doing amazing, I'm not worried about you."

Unintentionally I blurted out "Yeah - I don't want to be around this constant screeching, I'm handing my notice in today."

I went to the doctor's appointment as scheduled. I explained about the numb feelings, pinching my legs to demonstrate the lack of sensation. She decided the surgeon had probably damaged a nerve when he had operated. I also mentioned about the clinic and what they had said about my miscarriage. She sent me to the loo with a sample pot. I'd been desperate for a wee since I got there but hadn't wanted to miss my name being called. I proudly handed over my freshly prepared warm sample.

She left the room briefly and then returned beaming "Congratulations you're pregnant."

Whoa…Those were not the words I was expecting to hear; I wasn't even a grown up.

3

My State of Sobriety

Sometimes life takes a different path to what you had in mind. Travelling the world and partying into the early hours were put to one side; for now, anyway.

My mum hasn't had the easiest life. Hers was and still is, a cornucopia of anecdotes and chronicles but they are her stories to tell. She, perhaps unknowingly, makes the best of bad situations. She's had to - she's a mum. When I became a mum I also discovered my rose-tinted glasses.

My wonderful and unexpected surprise was nearly two years old. My boy and I had just got our first place - a maisonette above a little shop, located in the middle of a council estate overlooking a pub. The pub's clientele was not the sort that you'd particularly want to meet in a dark alley (or the bottom of the stairwell for that matter). Despite that, I painted the walls and filled the house with love and way too many toys. His dad and I were still young and neither of us had scripted a baby into our early chapters. We were good friends and he still made me smile so I kept trying to make our relationship work and for us to have the perfect family.

At first, I thought I was being clumsy, dropping things, tripping over nothing and falling over on occasion. I'd make excuses to myself. It was quite possible that I was just tired as I was doing an intensive NVQ course. It fitted around childcare for my little man.

The course choice had been between Accounting and Holistic Therapies. Seeing as I'd got a D in G.C.S.E Maths, which I retook and got a high B, my self-doubt when it came to figures, had already been embedded. On the other hand, my mum had always grown a herb garden and as a child, my dad always got me to walk up and down his back – so Holistic Therapies it would be. Surely with that resume I was already half-way there?

The little man went off to nursery every Saturday for the whole day, whilst I happily studied the reflex points of feet, essential oils, or massage routines. This was when I became hooked on the "alternative" medicines. I was definitely one of the more mature students but my peers were pleasant and I even came across a keeper of a friend.

During the evenings I'd sit upright on my gifted, second-hand, dining chair doing my best to ignore the singing, shouting and bottle smashes from the pub below. I typed away on a refurbished computer I had managed to keep alive, fitting in all of my studying and case studies at night whilst the little man slept. I worked really hard in my roles of being a good mum and studying for college. It did often leave me feeling drained. One night, after he'd had his dinner and a bath, I'd sat and read "Daniel's Train." He loved trains and was very much a boy's boy, playing with trains, cars and diggers despite me offering alternative "girls' toys," such as dolls, in an attempt to be a cool mum. As I kissed his forehead and left his room I tripped over. Luckily he had gone to sleep quickly and noises didn't disturb him. I had made sure that was the case by always hoovering or washing up during nap times in the early days.

I patted myself on the back and smirked, well I would have if I hadn't just whacked my knee on the wall. I convinced myself I must have been just tired. Studying whenever he slept and doing case-studies during his daytime naps would make anyone weak. Then however, over the next couple of weeks, the falling became frequent - too frequent. I also lost my appetite, which was swiftly followed by the smell of food making me want to throw up and the week after, the smells did have that affect.

Holding onto the pushchair to keep me upright, I headed to my doctors knowing that I couldn't ignore what was happening any longer. As I staggered into the surgery, wobbling and leaning all over the place, a middle-aged woman looked at me with disgust and shook her head, clearly questioning my state of sobriety. The doctor checked my ears and prescribed drops for what he assumed to be a common ailment; an ear infection which could have been affecting my balance. That week drinking (not alcohol!) became unbearable and made me vomit. I had abandoned my morning cups of tea and couldn't even sip water. I was losing weight too, technically most women's dream but I felt awful. Towards the end of the week, there was one night my body felt as if I had been run over, twice. I called the emergency doctors when the room started to spin. The out of hours' doctor prescribed Domperidone to try and halt the nausea. The next challenge came a couple of days later. It was so hard to see things through rose-tinted glasses when everything appeared blurry.

My little man was fantastic. He was in nappies and he adapted quickly to his rapidly aging mum. When he needed changing, he would come to me. I'd point at the bag of disposable nappies and he would toddle over and come back dragging the bag behind him. His little face lit up with a smile as he lay in front of me, keeping beautifully still, listening to my over exaggerated praise. I heard it too through my banging migraine.

He'd grown accustomed to my wobbly walks and was again, accompanying me to the doctors. My lack of focus and obligatory pushchair leaning stance probably still made me look like a drunk. I was fed up and demanded the doctor make me an emergency appointment. After phoning my partner to come and fetch the little man, I got a taxi and went to the hospital. My mum and Patrick would later be collecting him to stay with them in the mundane English countryside for a few days, just until I knew what was going on. The room was blurry and spinning more than usual. I was given a chair in the waiting area but I looked up and saw an empty bed which I climbed up on. At that point,

I discovered that when I lay on my right side and only my right side, the nausea lessened which gave me some relief.

I spoke to several doctors and after a couple of hours I was told I was going to be transferred to another hospital to run some tests. Another hour passed and I was approached by the hospital porter and he took me outside. The cool air felt amazing on the forehead of my pounding head before I was asked to climb into a minibus. I had to slump to my right, in my seat, to lessen the possibility of being sick on the journey. Every bump made me wince. The twenty-minute drive across town felt like a lifetime. We arrived and I was provided with a wheelchair while I waited for these "further tests."

I was then introduced to the MRI. The chap that wheeled me to the testing room asked if I minded if he came in. He'd always wanted to see what it involved. I felt so ill I probably would've agreed to anything. I climbed onto the unwelcoming plastic bed and was handed an emergency buzzer, which I was told to hold "just in case." Just in case of what? What were they going to do? They were going to insert me into the tube, which seemed okay, as I'd seen that in films and then they put what I can only describe as a Hannibal Lecter mask over my head to keep me still, with the instruction "whatever you do, try not to move." The room was still spinning round and round. All I kept thinking was "don't be sick don't be sick, if I move we'd have to start again. Don't be sick."

The noises, to anyone fortunate enough to not need an MRI, are a combination of whirly and chugging sounds. Perhaps similar to an electro rave on steroids? Eventually, after what felt like a decade of me repeating "don't be sick, don't be sick" to myself, I came out of the tube. "I feel sick and need to be sick." They handed me a tiny sick bowl.

"No, no I really need to be sick" and I ran out the room and across the hall into the toilet, swung the door open and just as it did, I projectile vomited. Almost seemingly like something from a scene in the Exorcist. The green forlorn porter said, "Is that normal?" Fortunately, they said it wasn't. I was put onto a ward and I lay there, in a big hospital bed, on my right side.

It was the birthday of my best friend from University. Only a trio of us had remained in the city after University finished, amidst the locals and new students that flooded certain parts of the town. We were the three musketeers. Musketeer number two came to sit with me after my other half had called her and I said "Happy birthday, you need to sort me out for the party - my eyebrows are horrid" laughing. My dedicated musketeer plucked away as I lay on one side. I couldn't sit up, so she fed me and helped me to sip my drink, which turned out in that position, was pretty difficult. I stayed in hospital that night.

In the morning the curtains were drawn around me and a doctor came in and stood next to my bed.

"Have you heard of MS?"

I felt a sinking feeling. My one experience of anything to do with that word, was of a lovely lady who was given that diagnosis and like so many before and no doubt many who followed, gave up. She was moved to a ground floor flat, got herself a wheelchair and rapidly declined. I had been sixteen at the time and used to harass her,

"Come on, we're going out for a walk."

She would get quite agitated at my persistence "I can't walk!"

"Come on. You'll be fine. I'll push you today."

"I don't want to go out, I've got MS I can't do anything. You don't understand," she replied.

"Have you heard of MS?" the doctor repeated, slightly louder this time. Maybe this was karma, I shouldn't have been so forceful. "It's not always fatal. A nurse will come and speak to you soon," and he walked away.

I moved the curtain back. The girl next to me smiled "Welcome to the club, it's not that bad, they'll explain. Really, you can carry on like normal, you just have to adapt slightly."

It was the Friday of May bank holiday so I sat and just waited. For what I'm not really sure. A part of me wondered if it was some epiphany of life and how it was a good thing that this had happened in order to make me a better person but three days sitting and just waiting, gives you time to think. Well actually it's pretty shit and unfair.

A nurse came with leaflets and said "If you've got any questions just let us know."

I smiled, "Will I get a disabled toilet key then?"

She burst out laughing, "I've never had that reaction before."

"Every cloud" I said, looking through my rose-tinted glasses. I was set up with a steroids drip. Little did I know but these would become my friend in the years ahead, as anyone else with MS will agree. I am so grateful to the girl in the next hospital bed.

I was sent home with an appointment for a home visit to teach me how to prepare and perform my own injections. Yes, that's right, injections to do by myself! They also gave me a date to attend a talk on MS and a visit to the local support group. Admittedly, my inner self rolled her eyes. I told musketeer number two (the birthday plucker) she had to come with me and hold my hand. We attended the talk in an extremely packed room. Most of what was said went straight in one ear and out the other. The only thing I recall is the woman at the front declaring that it wasn't genetic. I smiled and gave a huge sigh of relief. My little man wouldn't be affected.

The next trip was a dedicated support centre in the middle of an industrial estate. As we walked in, I noted the vast quantity of walking sticks, wheelchairs and people looking worn out as if regretting their last Sambuca shot. I wasn't like these people, I was fine as I thought to myself, "I'm never stepping in here ever again."

I was soon back home with my boy. I opened my post from that morning. There was a letter from the college stating that because I hadn't attended two consecutive lessons, I was being forced to leave the course. I was absolutely infuriated. I stormed into class on the Saturday and explained to my teacher about the recent diagnosis. She calmly said that she would speak to the head of the faculty and explain that all of my work was up to date and on medical grounds she would clear it. I loved my course that was originally just meant to be a bit of non-mummy time. The more I read about my topics, the more my thoughts were affirmed – there was more than just conventional science when it came to healing.

Luckily, they withdrew my expulsion. I'm sure there would have been some sort of disability discrimination claim if they hadn't but I was glad I didn't have to deal with that. I was in the twenty percent that passed. Many dropped out or failed assessments. It turned out that massage, reflexology and aromatherapy involved a lot more than just rubbing someone's various body parts.

The days, weeks and years went by. Having a child seemed to speed up time. I was getting more and more tired. The MS nurse (part of a small, dedicated team at the hospital) mentioned the use of a hyperbaric chamber - an oxygen chamber which apparently gave you a boost of energy - so I did it. I did what I said I would never do, I stepped back into that dedicated centre in the middle of that industrial estate. Everyone looked up and smiled. They still had the sticks and wheelchairs everywhere and people wobbling all over the place but I kept my thoughts firmly fixed on "I'm just going to use the chamber."

It was how I imagined being in a submarine. Ironically, you sat in an aeroplane seat without a seat belt, along with around five others. The operator placed my oxygen mask over my nose and mouth with the elasticated straps to hold it in place. It could take longer if you had to un-twirl the elastic from your hair or loosen the straps to allow blood to still flow around your face.

The operator spoke over a tannoy which caused me to slightly smirk, as he was only about 30cm away on the outside of the chamber.

"We're going down to pressure, let me know if there's any issues."

I kept swallowing and holding my breath, much like on an aeroplane flight, to stop my ears popping. I would later discover that this can be incredibly painful if you were due to get a cold.

Before I went into the crazy submarine, my wrists had felt like they were held tight with elastic bands. After an hour and a half, the operator told us we were going back to normal pressure. As I stepped out and removed my oxygen mask, I noticed the bands around my wrists had been removed too. Hang on a minute, perhaps there was something in this? Maybe I might return to this specialist centre in the middle of this industrial estate next week.

I did this and every week after for several years.

4

Not a Samurai

The most unwelcome of days had arrived; self-injecting 101.

The nurse came to see me complete with needles, medication and a lovely little, blue gift box for storage. She also brought along a firm foam sponge to practice my technique on before the real event and she gifted me a demonstration DVD for my viewing pleasure.

I could take my injections anywhere I wanted and I had a choice of injection sites. Hurrah. Thighs, arms (bring on the bingo wings) or stomach. Unfortunately, it had to be on my own body. The best and least painful place, apparently, was to inject in the stomach. The idea of this absolutely horrified me. All I could picture was myself on my knees, injection held tightly in both hands and…uggghh! Hara-kiri was not something I'd ever been tempted by. The stomach was, therefore, immediately ruled out.

I sat politely, taking deep breaths and admittedly, sweating in fear, as the matter-of-fact nurse showed me how to mix and prepare my injections. This reminded me of being in science class at school. Following her lead, I inserted the syringe drawing up the miraculous MS banishing clear fluid to blend with the other equally boring clear fluid. I was hoping for glitter or at least a change in colour - but nothing. The most exciting bit was a gentle flicking motion on the syringe to bring air bubbles to the top. After a quick practice stab of the foam with a faux injection, it was then my time to shine. My palms got sweatier, my breathing faster and after several huge swallows, I plunged the needle into my left thigh. The positioning was much more thought out than it may come across. I was to do this procedure every other day. I imagined noughts and crosses drawn on my legs as it wasn't recommended to do the same spot twice in a short period of time. I presume it's something to do with scar tissue and healing but to be honest, I try not to think about it too much. I was suddenly grateful for my thunder thighs - more flesh and ample spaces to choose from. The joy!

The unfazed lady left me with details of the company who would regularly deliver my goods. Then she proceeded to warn me about common side effects. These included fever, chills, joint pain, feeling unwell, sweating, headache, muscle pain and reactions at the injection site. Really - this would be something I would be inflicting on my body EVERY OTHER DAY?

When the morning of injection day came, I would pace around and keep myself really busy. I had so much that needed to be done first. Clearing out the kitchen drawer, cleaning the toys in the toy box, folding towels, pairing socks...or at least I would find things to be done.

Another site that was ruled out, at a later date, were my bingo wings. I'd mixed the injection, ready to go and held up my fleshy arm. My partner inserted the needle but slipped. This carried the needle in a most unwanted direction and was an altogether sickening experience.

I started noticing rashes. They appeared anytime I was prepping for my injection. At my next, now routine Neurology appointment, I discussed how stressful I found the regular self-harm activity. He also seemed unfazed - well of course they were unfazed, they didn't have to bloody stab themselves. He switched me to a weekly injection. It was a bigger needle but I only needed to puncture myself once a week - amazing.

I learnt quickly to rule out the day after my injection. Without fail, I'd wake up shaking and my muscles ached like never before. This was a minor sacrifice for one weekly injection. Mondays became the no go day. I figured Friday and Saturday nights I could play normally, inject on a Sunday, then do and be good for nothing on the Monday. I had to keep the injections in the fridge, so my tiny fridge began to always look fully stocked. Admittedly half of it was pharmaceuticals but full nonetheless. Yay for the second medication.

Day by day things were tough. My legs were sore climbing up the stairs to our house with the pushchair. I bought a fold up stick for the extra difficult days but was too embarrassed to use it. My best friend who lived round the corner would go to the shop underneath our home and bring up to the house what I needed. Milk, bread or more importantly chocolate. We had met at a toddler group before I had been tarred with the MS brush. After two sessions I decided I wanted to keep her. All the other mums were polite and kind but conversations of wet wipes and nappies grew tiresome fast. She was different, we spoke as women not mums and it was a welcome breath of fresh air. Perhaps ironic in a room full of dirty nappies. She told me about a get fit group she went to and invited me to join her. I decided that I would go along too. I got stronger and fitter as I lost my baby belly and felt like I was back at Uni with my gym bunny attitude. We were always the ones scoring the winning goals – top-of-the shop-first-over-the-line and became each other's advocates and healthy competition.

The instructor Nicole took the weekly fitness class and became my personal instructor as part of a government incentive scheme for mums. She was super fit and fun too, which spurred me to get back into exercise and weight training. Nicole met me at the gym once a week and was looking towards training me and my healthy competitor up to become fitness instructors. It sounded like a great opportunity. It was beep test week; Nicole, my healthy competitor and about ten other ladies were all lined up at one end of the hall. Beep. Run to the other side. Beep. Run back.

This continued and the beeps got faster and those that couldn't keep up dropped out. The beeps got closer together and soon there were only four of us still going. Nicole was at the side screaming encouraging words loudly. Another two ladies sat, bright red, panting and sweating. Beep. Just me and my favourite advocate left now. Beep. No way was I going to let her win, no way. Beep - level 9, she dropped. It was just me left with Nicole screaming "come on Kez!"

I remember thinking "two more beeps and that's me done." I made it! I went and gave my advocate a massive, sweaty hug. "All I needed was to beat you" and I winked.

"Well done lady" she said smiling.

From that point on my healthy competitor was known as Number 9.

Little did I realise only a few years later that it would be Number 9 carrying my bags and holding me up so I didn't fall. We were out shopping, I was using walking poles, moving slowly and she was carrying my basket. I ushered her to come sit with me as I couldn't walk anymore. I leant over and said "I still beat you on the beep test though."

"I know," she smiled.

I have to remind myself often of the stories of my fit and healthy body in the fear that if

I don't maybe my brain will forget.

During one of the later sessions with Nicole I was on the vertical climber. Nicole was shouting "come on Kez – you're nearly there!"

I panted back, red faced but still going "I can't feel my legs." Thinking it was just muscle fatigue, which any normal person would.

She yelled "That's good, you can't feel the pain!"

The three of us signed up for the race for life. We did loads of training together and our weekly group decided to challenge ourselves to an assault course. My friendly competitor number 9 and I, were under the nets caked in mud, then it was onto the tyres. I was just in front of her as we both sprinted to the climbing wall. I made it to the top. The zip wire was next before a short run to the finish. Looking down I just froze and stared. She was there a few seconds later. "Go Kez go!"

I just looked at her "I can't."

She just stared "you've done this before just hold on."

"I can't, I don't know why?" I said feeling scared.

She persuaded me to take the bar and pushed me off. I trusted number 9.

The moment took me back to when as a child, I'd been so excited at my first "proper" bike ride, which happened to be at breakneck speed whilst doing a circuit of the car park, with my family and neighbours watching on. To brake the ride, I'd flung myself to my right and crashed into a bush. I'd stood proudly brushing leaves and twigs from my hair with a massive grin on my face. My mum rushed over, looking concerned.

"How good was that?" I exclaimed.

My auntie sauntered over and looked at me "what's wrong with your brakes?"

"My what?"

When teenage years hit I always met up with my dear school friend in the morning, pre-school, occasionally applying my makeup first if there was a boy I liked. She was so pretty and amazing with makeup and she always made it look natural so we didn't get into trouble. We cycled together every morning.

The cycling continued as I got older and started going out into town. Whilst at college, everyone my age was desperate to learn how to drive and they asked for lessons for their Christmas and birthday presents. I didn't get it. I had a bike and this was my preferred and trusted companion.

Older still, I would cycle to the pub and then

cycle home. Only once did I get stopped for drunk driving by a beat bobby. I smiled, apologised, then walked for a bit before I jumped back on and cycled the rest of the way. I'd cycle to work too. Driving always seemed like an unnecessary expense to my pocket and the planet.

"What about when you have kids?" friends would ask.

"I'll teach them to cycle too."

My unexpected surprise learnt to cycle when he was around three years old - he was a natural. We cycled everywhere and had long cycle rides out to search for pirates and discover treasure by crawling through bushes. We'd also go shopping and I generally had a rucksack on my back and both handlebars would be laden with carrier bags. My little man started with an apple in a carrier bag swinging from his handlebars. It was after around the third shopping trip that he didn't moan about it being awkward. After that we gradually progressed to a rucksack. Now incidentally, he carries all the shopping, mostly.

As it happens, fate had bit me on the bum with my MS diagnosis. Despite my best intent, I succumbed to driving lessons when my surprise turned five. I was recommended a fabulous instructor by a girl from the MS centre; an animated Jamaican gentleman. I discovered that driving was better with music on, however, my left leg would sometimes just sleep. "What about automatic?" he suggested.

My partner and I had talked a lot about driving. Cars were not something I was remotely interested in. It was pointed out to me that if I learnt in an automatic, I would never be able to drive a manual. "Besides that," my partner said, "the mobility car we have is manual. Perhaps a different instructor would be better?" He recommended his former instructor.

About one out of every three lessons my left leg wouldn't play. Around the tenth lesson I became a bit teary.

"Let's pull over and swap." My driving instructor was thankfully understanding. "How about automatic? Its only to make sure you can get from A to B - you don't like cars anyway," he said in his unusual Aussie accent.

"I can recommend someone," my driving instructor suggested.

It turned out that this Australian chap actually came from Johannesburg and I wasn't the greatest at recognising accents. I deliberated a lot. Even my optician said he had an automatic. All the best and fastest cars were automatic apparently. I didn't want a car, of any sort, just legs that worked properly all the time.

I passed my theory and my practical test was soon after. I had been learning with the latest recommended instructor in an automatic. I sat there amongst swarms of anxious looking young people. A huge smiley man, one of the examiners, came out and I crossed my fingers. I felt my heart sink as he called out someone else's name.

A tiny scowling faced woman came out and called my name. I gulped. We went over to the car and I smiled at the examiner. As long as I didn't have to reverse around a corner, I would be fine. We got in and moments later we were off. I started chatting,

"You'll have to excuse me if I smell funny - I put rosemary on as it helps with memory. I was listening to a hypnosis on positivity this morning - I even eyed up my cat as I don't have a rabbit's foot." I laughed nervously at my own hilarity.

I could feel her stern look "I'd rather you concentrate than talk."

Rude cow.

"Now if you could just pull over to your left and reverse around this corner."

No, no, no I thought as I mounted the pavement, revved too hard and put my hand brake on. "Can we just head back to the test centre?" I begged.

We carried on for what felt like an eternity then headed back. I felt miserable, I didn't want to drive anyway. This was never a part of my plans. This was the first time I had had to admit MS had some power over me. I continued with my lessons.

The next time I was sat back in the test centre, I saw the huge smiley man again. He came out from a side room. I didn't bother crossing my fingers but when he called out my name, an equally huge smile spread across my face and I headed enthusiastically to my car. I didn't smell of rosemary this time but waffled on as nervously as before. He laughed appropriately at my spiel as we drove all around the countryside and eventually back to the test centre. I hadn't done a manoeuvre...

"Just park up in this bay for me."

But which one I thought, did it matter? "Any one" he added.

I parked, then drove back out and re-parked. "Shall I straighten up?"

Oh, so this was my manoeuvre. Eek.

"Whatever you think," his deep but soft voice said.

I didn't know, should I move? I pulled out then reversed again unnecessarily and put the brake on.

He got out the car and said he'd be back shortly. He came back and said "Congratulations, you can go on continuing to drive unwillingly and perhaps one day you'll like it."

Would it be wrong for me to propose to this man I thought and then I said it out loud.

He smiled warmly "Enjoy driving!"

5

Jellyfish

As a new driver, I was able to take myself to the dedicated centre in the middle of that industrial estate regularly. Just merely for oxygen of course. Whenever I'd been for a session I could tell the difference. The next day I would have much more energy than I usually had (or hadn't as the case was).

I remember being away on holiday for three weeks with the kids and their dad. After the first week I was exhausted but we weren't even half way through the trip. One day we went to a museum and we had just entered the foyer and I physically could do no more. I felt like I'd been hit by a bus - every inch of me hurt and my legs were not behaving like my friends anymore. I realised that a visit to the oxygen chamber was well overdue. I was clearly experiencing withdrawal symptoms.

It wasn't just MS sufferers, or MS fighters, as I prefer to say, that used the chamber. Famous athletes, speedway riders, footballers and the Leicester Rugby team were all regulars and they were all there for the precious oxygen. I was always oblivious to the famous people I shared the chamber with. It was only afterwards when another centre user would say "Wow, do you realise who you've been sat with?" I'd smile blankly and they'd explain.

The centre also offered different therapies and one being the group physio sessions. I decided I might go along and just see what the ill people were up to, I was fine after all. We sat round in a circle on our chairs. Some sat in wheelchairs, some with their sticks on the floor in front of them and then me, the fortunate one, who was absolutely fine. The physio that day was a Spanish lady, who was covering for the usual therapist. She started us off with neck rotations, arm stretches and shoulder rotations. These were done with varying degrees of proficiency and we gradually worked down to our feet.

"Just wiggle your toes everyone."

I heard the inevitable mutters of "I can't move

my toes."

She counted "one, two, three, fffff... someone count for me, I forget." She then pointed at a gentleman in a chair.

"He doesn't really speak" a voice said.

"Oh, I can try - one, two, umm, sorry my Spanish, I forget."

The non-speaking wheelchair man then, un-characteristically piped up "one, two, San tan der."

The room burst into laughter. The physio smiled knowingly.

As the class finished I asked the lady next to me as she reached for her stick "What medication do you take?"

She answered very matter-of-factly, "why - I have vitamin C every day."

Her general manner and happy air was contagious. She clearly wore rose-tinted spectacles.

I instantly knew she was a fighter and was going to be absolutely fine. In that one class, the ill people with wheelchairs, sticks and carers surrounding me became just people - and fighters who I admired. I started going to the MS centre regularly.

There were two complimentary therapists offering various treatments such as massage and reflexology. One of the therapists was about to go on maternity leave. The manager of the MS centre asked if I would cover. I happily agreed. After all, I had already started working as a holistic therapist at a little studio in town alongside one of the other girls in the 20 percent pass group. This would fit beautifully alongside that.

I started on two half days alongside my 20 percent pal as I had childcare to juggle and pay for. We both became busier with our workload and then she reached a point where she felt unsure which direction she wanted to take her business in. We decided to go our separate ways and I set up on my own.

I worked only a couple of days at the MS centre but loved every minute. It began to give me an insight into MS and the huge differences between how each person was affected but moreover, how they coped. Many of my "clients" and fellow MS fighters would tell me how much the treatments I gave would help them with their fatigue, stress levels, continence, muscle spasms and other symptoms. It gifted me a huge sense of worth. The centre users also gave me some incredible insights. One gentleman, a wheelchair user, gave me a piece of advice that I hold close to my heart, "don't be too stubborn to not use a wheelchair, but remember that once you get in, it's near impossible to get out."

My unexpected surprise was now six entire years old. My original life plan of not having my own biological children but to adopt, had certainly veered onto a different path. I had definitely watched too much Home and Away. There were too many children without homes and without people to love them. This all changed when my unexpected surprise arrived. I felt that bond that a child has with its mother. Although I was twenty-three years old when I had him, in my head I was still very young. I'd only just finished Uni and was still partying my weekends away. Despite many challenges that were thrown our way, myself and the little man did well and I learnt to become a mum.

Perhaps it was because my biological clock was ticking but I decided it was time to give the unexpected surprise a sibling. I spoke to his father, he was not so keen. He did not want any more children and reminded me that the neurologist had warned me that if I had any more children, I was likely to become ill, my MS would get worse. Now it may possibly be sexist, but only a woman understands the urge to have a child.

Life hadn't been easy, not that it ever is. The unexpected father and I had previously parted when my tummy was huge and then again when it had shrunk again. My surprise and I had done a fair bit of house jumping and it included a stay with one of my uni flatmates, AKA The Bakewell Tart, at her home near the sea. Three trains with a pushchair, a travel-cot and two bags loaded with bottles, nappies, toys and clothes for my bundle was no mean feat - and possibly a few pairs of knickers for me - I was a brand new mummy. At that point I didn't realise my little man would be fine as long as he had food, warmth and love. My Bakewell Tart by the sea had made up a big double bed for me with soaps, bubble baths, and chocolate lovingly left on the pillow. It was just what I needed. When she wasn't working, we went for long walks with the papoose on the cliffs overlooking the sea. She helped me blag my way to being a responsible mum. From there, we travelled to the other side of the country to the Fens and stayed with my young mum and Patrick Swayze.

I longed for the perfect 2.4 family, which kept me in a state of limbo wanting to be with the dad. The unexpected surprise and I stayed in a hostel but were eventually given a new home, the maisonette which we made into our first proper home.

After diagnosis, the stairs up to our home became impractical and were considered dangerous, so we were moved to a ground floor flat complete with a wet room.

His dad and I had finally reached a state of calm and tried again. I knew I was a strong woman, even though in my head I was blagging. He conceded and agreed to have another child. I carefully planned to come off my injections and started the washout period so that the baby would be "clean." Then I got pregnant quickly.

The Bakewell Tarts were staying over with us and one had already arrived. We sat drinking tea and reminiscing. She was and still is, a huge tea and toast fan. I, having drunk my weight in tea, went to the toilet and as I got up I looked down. There was a lot of blood. My heart raced. I walked into the living room, chewing on my thumb, my chest heavy.

"There's blood," I said as I pulled my friend into the loo, "that's not normal is it?"

She looked at me "That's a lot of blood Kez."

I went and explained to my partner. "There's nothing you can do." he said.

The three of us went straight to the hospital. I

turned to my friend, gulping back the tears, and said "I'm hoping it was twins and one is okay."

I had a frighteningly huge camera inserted into my nether regions and was told that my cervix was still closed. Did I dare breathe a sigh of relief? Later that evening I went back to the loo to be greeted with more blood. We went back to the hospital. At least I hadn't wasted my sigh.

Like many others, as soon as I'd discovered I was pregnant, I excitedly sent off for a free Bounty pack containing baby information and promotional samples. In this pack was tiny soft toy. To some this may seem inappropriate, but it's still safely stashed away in my attic, a small keepsake to this day. One in three pregnancies end in miscarriage. It's only because we are so technologically advanced that we even realise this cruel statistic. My way of dealing with it is that it just wasn't meant to be and this baby would've been quite poorly. I may have to deal with MS properly one-day people say, so a poorly baby as well may have been too hard.

A lot of persuasion with my partner to try one more time failed miserably. After an extremely drunken "life is too short" night out - I was pregnant again.

I was extremely careful with everything; half paranoia, half not wanting to be blamed for making it happen. At home with my little man and my tummy growing, I had an incredible pain. I was meant to be at work later but I cancelled my client. My boy and I got a taxi to the hospital. The doctor looked at me, "This pregnancy is not viable."

I looked in anguish, "it's going to be fine I know, please be careful because he doesn't know about this," I whispered to her, pointing towards my unexpected growing boy.

"It's not a viable pregnancy" she said again.

I rang their dad to come and collect our boy. I had a scan which revealed an eight centimetre cyst. The doctor told me it was dangerous and that they were going to cut it out.

I refused "I'll lose the baby."

Again she said, "This pregnancy is not viable."

I was getting angry now. "If you come near me, I will sue you and the hospital, I will sort it myself."

Realising she had a very difficult patient on her hands she backed down and discharged me with some medication to try and ease the pain. I sat, at night time, with both hands over the left side of my stomach where I assumed the ovary to be. I imagined lots of tiny jellyfish eating away at the cyst that was impossible to shift.

At my next scan, the cyst had shrunk to only six centimetres whilst my tummy was still growing. The next time it was four and a half centimetres cyst with my tummy still growing and blooming. Turns out that my imaginary jelly fish did me proud. I continued to grow and cycle to work daily until at eight and a half months, my huge tummy, void of any cyst, carrying my expected surprise, started crushing client's fingers as I leant over them.

I was doing everything right. I was eating well, avoided seafood, peanuts and all of the current recommendations. I attended aqua natal classes where I and other large-tummied mums-to-be, bobbed around in a relaxing pool. Afterwards, we discussed mummy type things over a drink. I also went to pregnancy yoga. Once a week planned bump and I, went and posed in strange positions in a room with other planned and unplanned bumps alike.

One morning, I'd dropped the little man off at school then went and bought some essential drain un-blocker. I collected the unexpected from school and left him with my partner before I sauntered off to yoga. Our instructor asked how we all were and when I said I might be in labour she laughed. A yoga mum gave me her pillow and I carried on with the class.

When I got in, we watched a horrifically troubling film about someone called Kevin. I stood up and felt that my back pain had increased. I thought a soothing bath might help. I was planning a water birth after all. I had my relaxation music all ready and organised and my oils blended for the different stages of labour. I ran the bath and as I started stripping off I felt a huge pain surge through me.

"Time to go!" I yelled.

We dropped off the unexpected surprise with his Auntie and headed straight to the hospital maternity wing. The pain had increased and was more frequent and I'd undone my seat belt to try and make myself a little more comfortable. By the time we arrived at the hospital I was leant forward on the dashboard in a very awkward position. I shuffled out of the car and instantly found comfort on my hands and knees directly on the car park ground. My partner went inside to be told there was no more room and that we would have to go to a different hospital. Sighing and grimacing, I got back in the car, not bothering with my seat belt and we raced through the city, possibly through several red lights in a rush to get to the next hospital. It was quite nerve racking as he had only passed his test two months prior.

We arrived at the next hospital – relieved to have arrived. The receptionist sent me straight into the assessment unit. I was asked what sort of birth I wanted.

"I wanted to have a water birth."

The midwife then wanted to assess me; I climbed up onto the bed and instinctively got on all fours. She looked and said, "I don't think we've got time for a water birth."

"Could I have a bath?" I counter offered.

"I really don't think we've got time" she replied.

Seven entire minutes, a lot of wincing, teeth clenching and what I can only describe as mooing noises later, the planned surprise arrived. I looked out of the window to a dark sky high-lighted with a beautiful splattering of twinkly stars. I glanced down at my expected surprise - she was beautiful. Her big brother was going to adore her, in small doses obviously. Luckily, she wasn't a boy, because if she had been, I had been told to put her back.

A lady knocked on the door "Congratulations - sorry to intrude but I saw you had a sticker to say you would donate your cord blood."

I filled out some forms and the lady went away beaming. I picked up my flip flops, then the new daddy and I left. "What's she called?" the receptionist asked.

"She's too good for a name, she may have a symbol," I laughed.

Less than five hours after giving birth, I was sat on the couch breastfeeding my expected at 6.30am, her big brother playing on the floor in front of us.

I had my 2.4 life now and my rose-tinted glasses were sat comfortably on the bridge of my nose.

6

Plasters and Pub crawls

My 2.4 home life was busy. We'd already bought a house together which needed a bit of updating. Plumbers were doing the bathroom, while further builders and tilers were doing the kitchen. It was all go.

My little man was now a lively seven-year-old. My young mum and Patrick had moved nearby to help us out. Unfortunately, their new house had fallen through so for now they were staying with a family friend. The house had no doubt become claustrophobic with all of them liking their own space and they would often pay an impromptu visit to our place; me, the young man, the little lady, our cat, six chickens, two plumbers, a team of builders and two tilers too. I learnt quickly how to multi-task breastfeeding and tea making. At first the workmen were shocked. They turned a bright shade of red and panicked but had to get over it quickly, if they wanted a supply of hot drinks and biscuits. My partner was working shifts and so, baby in hand, boy at side, I dealt with the guests and workmen.

I started getting increasingly fatigued and occasionally my eyesight would go blurry. This felt uncomfortably familiar, so I rang the neurologist but wasn't able to get through. The nurses had said it was early days. I started feeling quite ill and rang the neurologist often as everything became so hard. I left unanswered messages with secretaries and I became an irritating patient. They were probably thinking that I'd been warned but if we didn't do something fast, my body wouldn't be able to deal with what was happening to it. That night, when the kids had gone to sleep, I went to the fridge. As I opened the door the light came on and there it was. Sat there on the shelf was a left-over injection from months before. Surely that might help? I was desperate so I mixed it up and stuck it into my thigh. If I'd have known the facts, I would have realised this was pointless. The drug was cumulative and not a quick fix.

The days grew longer and my smiley babies kept me going between bangs and drilling, tea making and visitors. The kitchen was coming together so it wouldn't be long before we could cook. The toilet was plumbed in, so I didn't have to bug my neighbours anymore or persuade my first born to go in the garden. I ached all the time now. Perhaps Mike Tyson was sneaking over in-between that damn drilling and giving me a beating? One day it all felt too much for me and I reached tipping point. My eyesight was blurring again, I was dizzy, nauseous and lethargic and felt awful. I was promptly driven to the hospital's A and E department.

I was seen by an on call neurologist who said he would be dealing with me. Turns out it would be several years until I'd see him again. It was clear that I needed steroids and I asked them to book me in for a steroid infusion. They didn't have enough space for a private room for that procedure, and as the baby was only nine weeks old, they couldn't justify separating us. Instead, they prescribed me oral steroids which I took and left the hospital. I had to stop breastfeeding as steroids aren't great for little people, or adults come to that if over a long period of time. Despite only having a rather poxy amount of largely ineffective steroids, I had to carry on as any mum would. My partner was at work so I did the school run. It was cold and halfway to school, we had to stop as my legs were so sore. I finally dropped off my little man and went to nip to the loo before I walked back. The toilets were locked and the bell had gone - I'd just have to wait until I got home. I started the journey back, which realistically wasn't that far but on this day, it seemed a particularly long stretch. My legs felt heavy and grew tired quickly and then it started pouring down with rain.

That morning I hadn't been able to find the rain cover for the pushchair before we left and as we were going to be late, we left without it. To protect the little lady, I took off my coat and lay it over the top of the pushchair. The rain began to pelt down fiercely so I removed my glasses and put them safely in my bag. By this point I was leaning heavily on the pushchair for much needed support. My left leg had grown tired and I was dragging my foot along the ground. Several rest stops later and much wetter, we arrived home. Where were my keys? The little lady started crying, I scrambled through my bag, starting to get very agitated- where were they? Her screams loudened and the rain grew heavier. I had a mad panic as I was so desperate for the toilet. Surely this wasn't going to happen? Rummaging further I found my keys, still squinting with rain in my eyes. Now where were my glasses? I frantically tried to put the key in the door but it wouldn't open. Then it happened - something that everyone dreads.

When we eventually got into the house I stripped off my bottom layer, sorted myself out and grabbed some joggers. I quickly put them on, made up a bottle of milk and sat with my baby girl, comforting one another. I felt deeply humiliated but so grateful that no one else was there to witness what I prayed would be a one off. The morning school runs became harder still, then they became near impossible, then they were just that. Their dad did the morning school runs when he was on late shifts and my young mum and Patrick covered the others - this wasn't part of the 2.4 plan. I felt useless and redundant; I couldn't even take or collect my son from school – therefore, in my eyes, I was not a good mum.

The house was finished and looked fabulous but by then, I struggled to stand for any amount of time. Our dinners were focused around microwave meals or beans on toast. Long gone were the days I mocked packets of pre-grated cheese and pre-packed salads: they were a godsend. The new toilet and bathroom were gorgeous with a marble effect that reminded me of a Mediterranean style of decor. Truth be told, the stairs up to them became higher and steeper for me as the days passed.

One afternoon, the little lady had just eaten and had dozed off. I went to the bottom of the stairs and stared up at what seemed like Mount Everest. I took the first two steps but then my left leg wouldn't lift - I didn't get it. I lifted my dead leg using both hands to reach the next step, then stepped up. Still my leg chose to sleep. I grabbed the material of my trouser leg and wrenched my leg to the next stair and then stepped up with my other leg. My little lady started crying, but I was halfway to the loo. Surely she would settle down again. I managed to get myself near to the top of the stairs and it happened again! I was thirty not an old lady. I sat on the step like a toddler who'd had an accident. Embarrassed and ashamed - my silent tears shadowed my daughter's screams. I sat back down and bumped slowly down each step. That was uncomfortable anyway but this time my trousers were sodden. No one would need to know about this unfortunate incident, neither of them.

Things got even tougher. Their dad who'd been at work all day, would come home to a screaming baby daughter, an excited son with tales to tell and questions to ask and lastly, his girlfriend. Her appearance could be described as the following;

stir-crazy, hair never done, dishevelled, usually covered in baby drool and looked permanently exhausted. No freshly made dinners ever greeted him and although she tried to keep on top of the laundry and the washing up, her legs would just give way. Silent tears fell more frequently. I had a gorgeous home, a perfect little boy and baby girl and I didn't even have to inject myself. So why were my rose-tinted glasses so dirty?

I spent the days longing to go out and longing to do some "normal" stuff. When the little ones' dad got home, we'd drive out somewhere, usually to a park. I would perform my well-rehearsed pushchair lean, dragging one begrudging foot along with frequent stops to pause. When we were out, my little man had the opportunity to run around and let off steam. I felt alive but my left leg did not. My body became less willing to play, full stop. I couldn't do school runs, I struggled around the house and I wasn't breastfeeding because of the steroids. I felt like such a rubbish mum and an even worse housewife. Just standing was so hard – it's hard to comprehend unless you've been in that position I guess. After about a year, the neurologist decided it was time to try a new drug. I also received a referral to the continence clinic - bladder and bowel issues are massively common with MS. These referrals, although necessary, removed any remaining remnants of me being a desirable partner.

Tysabri was the next drug I was introduced to. Firstly, I had to sign a consent form confirming that I understood the increased risk of contracting a brain disease called PML. This trivial sounding side effect turned out to be Progressive Multifocal Leukoencephalopathy. One third to a half of those with PML die in the first few months. The odds however seemed in my favour, maybe? What other option did I have anyway? My cannula was inserted. I was one of only a handful that didn't even flinch at the needle, after all, I'd spent years doing my own.

The infusion was done at the hospital. It was always the same hospital, on the same ward and in the same bay, so I opted for the same time too. A nurse would come and ask me a few questions beforehand to make sure I was who I said I was. After all, I'm sure people swarm to be in with the chance to have a drip attached, especially with those odds! I would sit for an hour whilst the goop went into and circulated around my blood stream, followed by an hour to make sure I didn't have any major side effects or pass out - I guess that's why anyway. I drove to the hospital monthly - a necessary evil.

Everything in my schedule was planned around infusion dates. The nurses became friends and I got to know other patients and their stories too.

My legs got stronger, the washing up got done and basic meals started being prepared. I even started back at work and felt great. I signed up at a gym and started swimming regularly. The tread mill and weights weren't within my reach but I found a great yoga teacher. Life was back on the right track so I polished my rose-tinted glasses to remove the misery that had gathered. I took over all school runs, now by car not foot and worked the opposite shifts to my partner so that childcare wasn't an issue. Sometimes I'd work late but I would always creep into my babies' rooms to kiss them goodnight as they slept. I had the only car, so often I would drive their father to work, drop off the boy at school, take the little lady to my young mum's and then I would treat a client. After the client, I'd collect the girl, my boy from school, my partner from work, then I'd go back for another client. Life felt good, I had the perfect family, a gorgeous house and a job I loved.

I had to drive everywhere so I was eternally grateful to the huge smiley examiner. As the little lady had started walking, she often didn't want to be in the pushchair but I needed it. I persuaded her to hold on so we could walk together for as long as

I possibly could. The bus stop at the end of the road had moved to an impossible distance and it had become easier to drive to the supermarket. They had more choice anyway, surely?

"Why can't we walk today? It's sunny," the kids would sometimes ask.

I stopped coming up with excuses and just told the kids "mummy's legs don't work as well as they should."

Life ticked on as my rose-tinted glasses sat well on my face.

I'd drive and collect number 9 to go shopping. I clung to the trolley as if it were a pushchair. We went round the aisles picking my groceries, occasionally stopping. If my legs refused to move, we'd pretend to be deep in conversation or be admiring a product on the shelves. If I were feeling really adventurous, we'd venture into town. I would hold number 9's arm and occasionally had to use the stick as well in the other hand. We frequented many a café, sometimes for breakfast, sometimes lunch or just for tea and coffee. These outings kept me feeling normal. As the weeks, months and years passed, the outings became less as I would trip over my own feet. The stick was now fully on show and its use could no longer be disguised. Number 9 always made me smile. When I stumbled she would catch me before I hit the ground but offered to throw herself down to distract attention if she didn't catch me - she always caught me. We met up once and she had handmade the most fanciful plasters "so we can celebrate the falls," she said.

Many people went out on pub crawls. I used to love going on pub crawls. One of my theatre friends, the third and final musketeer, had suggested we go out drinking, for old time's sake…I smiled at the thought but knew it wasn't a possibility - I couldn't even walk to the shop at the end of my road. "We'll get taxis, come on," she urged.

Seeing her always brought back memories of us dancing through the night and laughing – we were always laughing. We got dressed up – ish: I had gotten rid of any clothes with buttons as I couldn't do them anymore, they were far too fiddly. I didn't wear earrings or bracelets, necklaces or anything that required any amount of dexterity. My shoes were all flats and I had elasticated waists so to prevent previously undisclosed events. I threw on a dress over my head and went without make-up. Shaky clown-like makeup wasn't in fashion, nor bloodshot eyes from stabbing myself with an eyeliner pencil. I wasn't a big one for make-up anyway.

Our taxi arrived and we were off, arm in arm and stick in hand. On arrival at the first bar, she ran ahead and bagged the table closest to the door. I clung to the wall willing my legs to make it up the two steps - I made it! We sat and laughed as if without a care in the world. Then she ushered me away. "We're on a pub crawl, aren't we? Come on, let's go."

She then hailed a taxi outside and asked him to drive to the next bar at the top of the street (about 200yards). He laughed at first and then got angry "You are kidding me, right?"

My musketeer did not give in and fought for my honour "Are you a taxi driver? Surely you're not refusing a customer request. Is my money not good enough?"

Rightly enough he drove us there, she overpaid him but refused any money from me. "I asked you out," she said sternly, she meant business.

We sat and drank in that pub and then the one next door. We drank too much and laughed even more.

7

Smudge on my glasses

Tysabri did what it was meant to - slow the inevitable progression of the MS.

Years passed and life was good but had just altered slightly. I drove everywhere, not out of choice but it allowed me to be able to go shopping, keep working, socialise and most importantly, play mum.

The first time I couldn't do the school run it broke my heart. A trivial and simple thing that people take for granted. With the help of the school, who had given me a pass so I could drive right up to the building, I was able to play mum again. Admittedly, I wasn't volunteering to help on school outings and certainly not with the P.E. lessons like I had with my son. I was using a stick all the time but I could still sit and make Christmas crafts with my little lady. I wasn't missing those magical moments for anything.

My clothes were all elasticated and my shoes were either slip-on's or had Velcro-fastening so they were easy to get on and off with my now decreasing dexterity. I scarcely wore jewellery and was void of make-up, I bought ready prepared and chopped food. Now I may not have been Nigella but our meals were no longer a choice between baked beans or microwave food. Unfortunately, on a couple of occasions, a combination of poor motor skills and lack of sensation ended up giving me a sharp shock; well more of a slow burn actually. I'd been leant forward in the kitchen with my weight on my left hand, whilst hacking away with a knife in the other. A moment and an unpleasant burning smell later, I realised my left hand was frying on top of the hot hob. The normal pain response just hadn't registered. Tripping over thin air became a frequent activity and I dropped most things. I stopped going to yoga as I struggled to stand, let alone do the poses. Any trips out were planned around distances from the car park, avoiding having to go up too many steps and of course, having a loo in the nearby vicinity.

I had already been referred to the Continence Clinic but the next referrals were to an Occupational

Therapist, a Physiotherapist and the Gait Lab. My bowels were good but it seemed my bladder was not in correlation to a woman of my age. It's understandable for old ladies to piss themselves. It's widely accepted for toddlers to piss themselves. It was not acceptable for me in my thirties to piss myself. The advertising of certain brands, were sold to us by smiley women playing tennis, but it was not so smiley for those needing to buy the actual products. They were the items you did your best to hide in the bottom of the shopping trolley.

The Occupational Therapist was available to offer advice and help me cope with everyday living. She was positive, encouraging, understanding and kind. She wasn't judgmental or patronising in any way. This fantastic woman taught me tricks to enhance my dexterity and sensation, such as hiding small items in bowls of pasta. The idea of this strange sounding activity was to develop motor skills and sensation. Differentiating between the pasta and other items may seem easy but when your sense of touch is akin to wearing a thick pair of mittens. In one session, a couple of tears escaped as I opened up, feeling guilty about how I had to impose on others for everyday things that I should be doing myself.

Physio was in some ways like yoga. I was not

to be comparing myself to others but just to myself. 'You're older now' I tried to convince myself. Yeah, about a year older at most. The cruellest part of MS is that it takes things away slowly, so you don't realise the deterioration taking place. You alter things around you to adapt them to suit your needs but then suddenly they are an impossibility.

My physiotherapy sessions at hospital became an unwanted event. I was once told to sit on a yoga ball and raise my leg. I tried to explain that my balance was poor and that I'd probably end up on my bum. The physio was persistent. I raised my leg then lo and behold I fell to the floor. Fortunately, that set of Physio sessions ended shortly after. I'd already taken exception to the therapist but luckily they usually work on rotation, so another referral would more than likely be with someone else.

It was the summer holidays and we were going to go with family to visit other relatives in Germany. We, being the kids, their father, their grandpa, their aunt, their two cousins, a girlfriend and me. It was a wonderful group and fortunately we made each other laugh, a lot. As both the kids' father and grandpa were petrified of flying, travelling by train was going to make for a long journey.

From the start, the children were swarmed with

people to entertain them. We set off. Everyone was great and carried my bags and tickets the whole time. The only thing I had to do was move myself - this was becoming more of a challenge. We firstly got the train to London. From London to Brussels, then to the first stop in Germany. Despite the necessary platform changes and connections, I felt optimistic that I could do it. All was good until we came to the last leg. Our train was just pulling into the station so everyone was running haphazardly in that general direction. It had already been a long day, I was exhausted and my legs weren't happy. The lift would be quicker than me having to raise my legs up and climb every step, one at a time, potentially with my hands. My eldest nephew was by my side at the base of the lift. We heard yelps from the others "the train's here run, run" at the same time many footsteps racing up the steps next to us.

My nephew was furious. His anger was overshadowed however by my feeling of guilt at being a constant burden. He spoke through gritted teeth staring straight ahead. "They're fucking out of order if they've left us, you're fucking disabled and I'm so fucking angry."

As the lift went up I had this horrid feeling in the bottom of my stomach. The lift doors opened as we saw the train doors close and then pull away.

The children's father stepped out from behind a pillar "We've missed the train; the kids are with the others."

We sat and waited for the next train with my nephew's irate interjections breaking up the atmosphere of my guilt and the dad's frustrated anger. We made it to the house, much later than everyone else obviously. The next day we all went swimming, it was a fantastic water park with the highest diving boards and long slides. Family members took it in turns to outdo each other not only on the height of the board but through their high diving prowess, which was in fact, mostly belly flops. It was great fun and although I wasn't diving, I had so many giggles with our family of many generations.

Afterwards we headed back to the house. I kept up with the rear of the group but after a while my legs grew tired and slowly my foot started to drag. The children's father stayed with me. We took several breaks and sat on walls to allow my legs to wake up but after about half an hour of doing this, my left foot just outright refused to go any further. I felt so guilt-ridden that all the family were probably now back at the house whilst he was sat on a wall in the boiling heat unable to go anywhere. I was just grateful it wasn't raining. In the end, he threw me over his shoulder and gave me a fireman's lift to the end of the street. He placed me down and I managed one step, but no further. I was ashamed at how humiliating this must be for him having to carry his partner down the street. "I'm really sorry," I said. He remained silent.

The next day, everyone went for a family walk while I stayed in with the great aunt. We drank peach Schnapps and laughed so much that the language barrier wasn't an issue. Later in the week, feeling optimistic and rested, we all took a slow stroll into the city centre…almost. I got so close and within reaching distance when my legs said no more. There wasn't any point going any further, I knew my legs wouldn't be playing and I couldn't slow everyone down, not again. Instead I'd sit at the table at a little coffee shop and drink tea. I had a good book, the sun was out and I liked tea. As the days advanced, I passed on other outings, instead drinking tea and alcohol with the great aunt. She went from a great aunt to a fantastic aunt soon after meeting her. I can vouch it wasn't the alcohol or pity on her behalf, we shared an admirable connection despite the language barrier.

A handful of our family were flying back to England instead of staying on longer. The children's father presented me with my ticket back. I had a Tysabri session so had to be back for that. The children, their dad and grandad were going on to Berlin and Cologne. Both were beautiful cities that I had fallen in love with on my first ever visit. The history that seeps from the very core of Berlin made my heart pound and the architecture of Cologne took my breath away and made me want to declare that I'd found my artistic soul. My legs hadn't allowed me to move and I had to go for my monthly infusion. It made sense but I was totally gutted. MS was proving people right - I couldn't do normal things like normal people anymore. The children's father often said to me that I needed to stay home and rest. He would take the kids out to run around and play. "Just stay home, let the kids be kids."

This statement often rushed around in my head. I still did their cooking, cleaning and washed their clothes and I wasn't trying to take anything away from their childhood. A familiar wave of guilt filled every single shallow breath I took. I was a rubbish partner, a terrible housewife and clearly a dreadful holiday companion but it was thinking I was a shitty mum that tore at my heart.

When I got back to England I'd be solo for two

weeks. I'd had a huge clear out before we left for Germany and planned to do a car boot whilst the kids were away. I had also been referred for more physio and had my infusion booked. I rang number 9; she knew how much I hated missing out. When we had first met, we talked about a girly holiday but it was always just a bit of a joke as neither of us could just up and go. "I'm heading back to go for my infusion, my legs aren't great, but do you fancy that girly holiday? I won't be able to do much, but we could sit and sunbathe maybe?"

She was enthused at my suggestion and then referred to an outing we'd had the year before. I was at the time, feeling worthless which is unfortunately a common MS theme. I joked at how I was jealous of joggers and was going to stick my leg out and trip them over as they galloped past me without a care in the world. I mentioned my envy of casual shoppers.

"Right, let's go," she exclaimed, "you wanted to go shopping so let's go to Nottingham."

By rail I wouldn't have been able to walk from the platform to the town centre with enough energy to potter, I knew my body was too weak. She ignored my droll tones and said

"Okay, you're driving."

I perked up - I did have a blue badge after all and surely that was the equivalent of a superhero cape, invisibility cloak or light sabre. I drove us to the centre of Nottingham and abruptly stopped the instant we found a car park and claimed our space. We walked about a hundred metres then sat and had a coffee and tea in the first café we came to. After that, we strolled to another café and it was at this point the glorious "Fuck It Bucket" was created. This was a hypothetical container that would hold all my negative "I can't do's," and it was at this point I left my "rubbish holiday companion" thoughts behind in the confines of that bucket.

I left Germany with happy thoughts of an anticipated girly trip. The flight from Germany was short, we landed back in England and got a train and relevant taxis to our respective homes. I filled my car and got up early the next morning and persuaded one of number 9's good friends to join me at the crack of dawn for the car boot. How could she refuse?

The very next day I had my scheduled infusion at the hospital. A few hours later, was physio - luckily with a new lady who didn't make me fall on my bum. Number 9, true to the 'fuck it bucket' ways, had booked us a holiday. Her husband collected me and my bag and dropped us both at the airport. Number 9 wheeled our bags and we were off to sunny Majorca! We purposefully booked excursions so that we would be collected from our hotel door. We walked to the beach, extremely slowly and with many a stop but we did it. As fate would have it, one of the many tacky beach shops happened to sell walking poles. Quite probably for the drunken Brits, after all, Magaluf was just a stone's throw away.

One of the excursions was a tour of historic Majorca and we found ourselves sat on a rickety old train which ran along the very edge of the mountain with a sheer drop. The views were pretty hair-raising. The train stopped for a photo opportunity and refreshments.

"For the ideal photo and refreshments, you simply have to climb the rest of the mountain" the guide chirpily announced in their Spanish accent.

"You're kidding me," I said – not believing my ears.

Number 9 smiled. "When have we ever turned back? Put climb a mountain in the bucket."

We did just that. Slowly, very slowly, but surely, we reached the top and took some great pics of the spectacular panoramic views and cooled down with a slushie. The next trip was out on a glass bottomed catamaran with the opportunity to go snorkelling. We sat sunning ourselves in our short-sleeved tops, straw hats and sunglasses. It was a boiling hot day and the cool breeze was welcoming. The boat stopped - snorkel time! I smiled at number 9, she looked unconvinced. The jump down into the sea wasn't a slight distance from the edge of the boat. I smiled "I'll go first for the fuc…" leaping into the air from the safe confines of the boat and into the sea.

When I bobbed back up, I wiped the stinging salty sea water and sun cream combo from my eyes, "…k it bucket," completing my sentence.

Number 9 took a deep breath then jumped in and joined me in the turquoise water.

A small group of us snorkelled and we saw the most beautiful fish swimming close to us. Then it was time to get back onto the boat. The waves were crashing against the boat and people swam up to the ladders attached to the sides. I could easily get hold of one of the string ladders, but it took me many attempts to lift my leg up, and number 9, despite the choppy waters, pushed me towards the ladder. My leg was really angry but fuck it - we did it! As the trip was coming to an end and nearing the shore, the crew produced a plank of wood. "We can't dock here so is everyone okay to walk the plank?" was sort of what was said in a broken English/Spanish combo.

As we "docked up" everyone rushed and crossed the plank to the land, leaving just me and number 9. I knew I looked scared now. The captain ushered number 9 to cross then crossed himself. Was I to be left to join the next group? The captain then walked back across the thin wooden plank and put his hands out to me. I took hold of his hands and one slow step at a time, mirrored him as he walked backwards until we were on dry land. As I re-visited dirty dancing again in my mind, I sniggered to myself.

The next sunny morning we took another snail's pace stroll to the beach. We saw a board advertising parasailing. "Do you fancy it?" Number 9 asked with a grin.

"Hell yeah!" I said, at which point number 9 swiftly paid.

I found out what parasailing was over lunch.

We rocked up to the beach the next day, well rocked is probably the wrong adjective, more like ambled. We then saw exactly what we had signed up for, oh my! They did a test to check our balance. I can't even remember how I fared but I obviously had an appalling result, so was placed in the centre of the boat with the other, equally less gifted on the balance front, soon-to-be parasailers. We were given huge life jackets to put on and once they were checked, the speed boat in front of us raced ahead. 'What's going on' I wondered before I was suddenly whooshed into the air like a rocket. It was the most exhilarating rush. As we floated in the bright blue sky, the ocean beneath us, I shouted over to number 9 "This is perfect for the bucket!"

I smiled to number 9 and thought to myself "Fuck you MS!"

8

The Situation

The week away passed so quickly but it was just what I needed. I felt strong, both mentally and physically. To be fair, the walking poles may have been responsible for making my movement so much easier. Our bags were fully laden with gifts and precious items such as shells, pebbles and some hotel jam. The miniature jars that just ask to be taken with you!

We'd both bought ourselves pretty ankle bracelets and agreed that when they wore out it would be time to book our next trip.

Number 9 and I walked through the airport,

both sporting huge sunhats that we'd purchased a few days earlier for the boat trip. I moved along briskly with the poles, number 9 following closely behind just like the old days. I was 9.2 on the beep test after all. In her defence, she was wheeling two massive cases which we were about to discover at check in, were very overweight. Oops. The man at the desk looked at us both, glanced back at the scales and shook his head. Although I'd like to say he let us through anyway because we looked so fabulous; tanned and parading our showy big straw hats, in reality, it was probably my sticks that bought us a bit of lee-way. Every cloud.

A short flight later and we'd arrived back from our holiday. The kids and their father would arrive a day later. Myself and number 9 had proven that I wasn't useless, that I was a good holiday companion and thanks to the fuck it bucket, I knew that if I put my mind to anything, I could make it happen. After all, we'd climbed a mountain, jumped off a boat to go snorkelling, walked the plank, (granted with the captain) and we'd been parasailing. Not your average sunbed-and-not-budge-for-a-week trip I'll have you know. My MS wasn't going to hold me back. It might make me adapt a few things but it was not going to control me. Number 9 had made me realise that - hashtag not on the scrapheap (#notonthescrapheap)! I was going to try my best to be a good housewife, a good partner and most of all – a brilliant mummy (even if I had a wonky leg).

The children's father jumped straight back into his shift work. He was going for a promotion and seemed quite stressed about it. He sat up late at night doing application forms and was also doing an online course alongside his job. In the evenings, after we put the children to bed, I sat and helped him with his coursework and application forms.

Shortly after this period, I clearly remember him suggesting again that he take the children out so they could have a run around and play, while I rested at home. I did need rest and a big part of MS is the fatigue. That said, I didn't want to rest all the time - I wanted to be a good mummy and I wanted to be a good partner. I didn't want to be the ill, disabled one that had to stay at home and rest all the time. Although that's probably what you're meant to do if you have MS, it was not an image I identified with.

Their father seemed to be on edge all the time. "He's probably feeling stressed with needing to earn most of the money to make ends' meet," I thought to myself. He would come back late from work and

I often suggested to him to go and meet up with his friends while I watched the kids. He deserved to have a night off after being busy at work all day. It must have been difficult for him; he had a full-time job and was coming home to children and a partner that was perhaps, still considered, disabled - I did have a wonky leg after all. The holiday I went on with number 9 gave me a new lease of life. I knew that I wasn't just the disabled person with MS, I was more than that. I could still be fun and I would make sure I was a good mummy and a good housewife. I'd keep on top of washing clothes and the dishes, I tried to cook dinners from scratch but standing would be difficult. I split the task into sections - firstly I'd sit and chop. Next, after a brief rest, I returned to finish off. Don't get me wrong it took a long time but I tried to provide better meals than just boring beans on toast. Sometimes I was just too exhausted though. I was probably not the most fun to be around I thought.

As the days, weeks and months went on, the children's father seemed to be distant. He was probably concerned about work and he started getting short with me. I thought he must be fed up - he was earning all the money after all. Although I tried to keep on top of it, the house wasn't always spotless.

Hoovering was exhausting and mopping was near impossible, I was convinced I was going to fall over. I did try my best but sometimes that just didn't seem good enough.

The car boot friend of number 9's had a cat that she couldn't keep any more. We'd had a cat several years before that the kids adored, but inevitably, like all pets, he passed away. I spoke to their father about taking in the cat, he refused saying it was too much hassle. I'd grown up in a fabulous house full of animals; four dogs, a cat, some budgies, a rabbit, a guinea pig and many fish. A cat is quite self-sufficient I tried to convince him. He was not to be convinced.

My not so little man overheard the cat conversation and begged me "please mum, please can we get a cat – please."

I just looked at their father. He said in a very angry voice "just do what you want!"

He was a man on the edge, struggling to balance work and home life with a disabled partner and he was clearly finding life frustrating. All of these are valid reasons, but ultimately, not a fantastic thing to come home to.

How ingredients finish up as a dinner and are

served nicely on a plate and laid on the dining table is irrelevant if you've been at work all day on a long shift. Now, their father was like most men, in the fact that his thoughts and feelings were kept locked inside. I have the irritating habit of saying what comes straight into my head out loud. I pulled him to one side, not literally - I wasn't about to fall over. I'd spoken to him often over the last few months and would ask if there was anything I could help with. Was he struggling at work? What did he need? It became quite apparent that he was not happy, which I could understand. Life doesn't always play out exactly as you planned.

One time he was sat in the garden with his head in his hands. A typical pose for a broken man. I put my left hand on his shoulder while my right hand held on to my stick.

"What can I do to make things easier for you?"

He just turned to me, eyes puffy "the difference is, I choose to be part of this situation, you don't have a choice - you have to be part of the situation."

I didn't really understand - what situation? Then it became quite apparent - the situation was the MS. I had no choice it was true but he did have the choice and he was still here.

Number 9 rang - the cat desperately needed a

new home. I looked at their father. "Do what you want," resounded in my head. I'd done nothing but try, so hard. I took a deep breath, put the inevitable conflict to one side, I told the not so little man to get into the car and we drove off to fetch the cat. Now I had been warned about this shaggy coated cat. I was warned "don't touch his paws and don't touch his belly, as he can be quite vicious." Was this a good idea? After all, I had two children. Well, we'll just see how we get on I thought. We took the big, fluffy ball of fur back to the house.

Christmas was less than a week away and this year we were giving the shaggy moggy a home. I love the build up to Christmas. We make decorations and put them around the house. Best of all though is the sparkly, lit up Christmas tree. Each Christmas Eve, my mum, the kids and I, make mince pies and sausage rolls, then later put food out for Santa and the reindeer.

The very next day, our 2.4 family went to the Snow Dome, a self-enclosed Christmas in its own right. We had our warmest clothes on. Heat and MS are not great together, the cold and MS affects me even more but this was a family outing.

"We haven't done this for such a long time." I said.

I put on tights and my thermals under my woollen leggings. Woolly socks were snug under my boots so I wasn't going to get cold. We were going to have the best day out together as a family. We stroked all of the reindeer's and trudged through the snow together. The kids took it in turns on the sled. The children's father suggested that I sit down and he pulled the sled around the snow with me chuckling as much as the kids.

I thought to myself, "Things are going to be alright, we're going to make this work after all. The MS. was not going to control me, I was going to control the MS. It was not going to ruin my family."

We even saw Santa - it was the most magical day. As all attractions do, they offered us photos of our wonderful experience and snow globes with our pictures on. They were of course all hugely overpriced, but I wanted to capture this day.

"Let's get the package," I said excitedly.

Their father just shook his head, "It's really expensive - we don't need to do that."

This was special. It had been an amazing day and this was going to be the first day of the rest of our lives. I was going to try my hardest. I was going to get stronger - I felt it in my head and so my head would rule my body. I would make my body stronger so that I could be a better partner, have a tidier house and most importantly, be a better mum. Their father had made a valid point - they were extremely overpriced and because I didn't want to cause an argument I just agreed. We got one photo to celebrate that special day but the memories were more important anyway I reassured myself.

On the drive home the children slept. I always have so much to say, so with my blathering on about Santa and the kids' faces, the snowball fights and the sledging, I filled what would have been in hindsight, an awkward atmosphere. It was only five days until Christmas and Father Christmas would be coming soon. We sat downstairs in the lounge and the kids were in bed. I smiled at their father,

"Ok?"

He just looked at me "I can't do this anymore."

"It's nearly Christmas," I pleaded, feeling my voice rise.

We were meant to all be having Christmas dinner with his family. I hadn't bought any food. "What can I do to make things right? How can I make you happy?"

"I just don't want to do this anymore," he insisted.

I took a deep breath, a lump firmly lodged in

my throat. I didn't have a choice and he did. The MS had won.

"I'm sorry I couldn't be there for you," he said, tears in his eyes.

"And I'm sorry I didn't appreciate you enough," I said with puffy eyes and a snotty nose.

With that he left. It probably wasn't the best visual of me, with my swollen face and snot dripping down onto my reddened cheeks. That night, I had the typical clichéd reaction that the best films have in these situations and I cried into my pillow. With an added difference, the shaggy rescue cat jumped up and sat by my head as if he could sense my sorrow. In the following weeks I discovered he would keep himself to himself but whenever the silent tears came, so did the cat. I used many different excuses to the children for why I looked teary and my eyes were swollen. My main one was that I'd been cutting onions. I realised shortly after, I needed to have some onions nearby at all times.

Christmas came and the kid's father had been staying away. I told him on Christmas Eve that he had to come back first thing in the morning so that the kids woke up with him at home. Somehow we had a proper family Christmas. He wanted to tell the children but there was no way I'd allow their little hearts to be broken then. I should have won an Oscar as we went and had a family dinner at his sister's. I smiled, I joked and even laughed in the right places. It was wonderful to see the whole family. My nephews and my "sister-in-law," were always very precious to me and always will be. At the end of the day, their father stayed. I drove home with the happy yet worn out kids, put them to bed and along came the silent tears.....and the cat.

9

The Uninteresting Man

I awoke the next morning with an unfamiliar and terrifying feeling I had never felt before, nor do I ever want to again. My whole body felt as if a heavy weight was pressing down on me and I felt like throwing up. Why did I have to wake up? My whole world was about to crumble in front of me. I had spent thirteen years as the cement that kept the family together. Any cracks I had smoothed over with smiles and laughter. Any holes I had stuffed with compassion, forgiveness and love. The MS was a huge hole but I thought over time I would fill that too. It's what I did.

Then I remembered my beautiful babies - my not so little boy and my little lady. I would never let harm come to them and would give everything I had to keep smiles on their little faces. The "She-Ra" was unleashed within me at that moment. What was to happen over the next six months is a story in its own right but it involved my badass "She-Ra" self and the biggest blag I'd mastered to date. As karma/god/fate, or my rose-tinted glasses would have it, I bought their father out of the house. It became ours and no matter what, this was going to be our sanctuary.

Shortly after Christmas a remarkable and inexplicable thing happened. I went for a cuppa and catch up with my young mum. She, alongside my silent tear cat, had kept my eyes dry and glasses tinted. We sat in the first café directly across the road from where I parked the car. I ordered us a huge pot of tea at the counter, paid and then, it happened. I carried the tray with the pot of tea, two cups, and two saucers, totally unaided across the café to our table. My young mum's face lit up - for the next few days, it was as if my body had been re-booted. I even managed to carry a Christmas diorama model up the stairs, without holding onto the banister. It is common knowledge that stress exacerbates symptoms in MS so what was this miracle?

Unfortunately, my body soon reverted back to

my clumsy, tripping-on-thin-air self. I struggled to get to the bathroom more than I will ever share. In secret, I visited the continence clinic. The clinician gave me some great news, which I held and still hold dear. My bladder control is brilliant and I can hold an exceptional amount of urine. Not sure if I will be making a placard to share this information though. The issues I was having were attributed to two things. Firstly, my fine motor skills, or lack of; undoing zips and buttons was nearly impossible. I'd dealt with this already by wearing elasticated clothing. Secondly, and much harder to remedy, was my mobility, or lack of. I was struggling to get up the stairs when the call of nature came. If my leg was refusing to work, I'd have to lift it with my hands, step by step, to get upstairs. I just couldn't move fast enough. After many chats with the team at the MS centre and with some of the regulars, it seemed there was help to be had in the form of adaptations to my home. Despite my initial reluctance to change anything in the house, I applied for a government grant. Maybe a teeny bit of help wouldn't go amiss.

I had an occupational therapist come to assess me and with a supporting letter written by the MS nurse, they both agreed that I needed easier access to the bathroom but also to my bedroom too. Whoa - I'd never even thought of that. Over the next few months, I had various interviews and visits and it was agreed that I was eligible for the grant. Someone from the council inspected the property and thought a lift being fitted would be the best solution. Now in theory this sounds great but when I looked at the designs, it was another matter.

The lift would go from my front room up into my bedroom. The lift needed to be large enough to fit a wheelchair and a carer, after all that was the inevitable outcome. As the lift required a large amount of space, we would only have just enough room for a small sofa or a couple of chairs in our living space. Now anyone who has squabbling kids will recognise that this would be a cruel thing for any parent. There'd be me and both kids having to share the sofa. In my bedroom there would only be space for a single bed. Now I realised I couldn't wear makeup or jewellery and that I lived in elasticated clothes - but no wardrobe? I WAS STILL A WOMAN for fucks' sake.

The bathroom was to be transformed into a wet room, with the doorway extended to fit my wheelchair through. Fine, but I didn't have, nor was I going to end up in a wheelchair. At one of the interviews I was asked how I got up the stairs at the moment. I feel I may have shot myself in the foot, but I openly explained how I would just sleep on the sofa if I was too tired. For these times I explained that it would make things easier to have a toilet downstairs.

Along came occupational therapist number two. He was of the opinion that I could and should sleep downstairs in my front room. In fact, we would design it as an all in one. A single bed and shower cubicle about a metre apart, with a toilet placed neatly within! Can you imagine that scenario? I was to sleep in the same room as my toilet. Okay so that's far from ideal but shit, where I washed also? Surely this was a joke. The continence issue was humiliating enough as it was but this highlighted the fact that I was a woman in her 30s who was different from everyone else. Every child is embarrassed by their parents but this would make mummy different. Hell, I was embarrassed by me. Financially, this was a better option for the decision makers. I argued that it would put boundaries between me and the children and that we needed family space but was repeatedly told this solution ticked all the boxes.

Needless to say I was not impressed at their proposition. After numerous enquiries I found out about an equivalence grant scheme. The money that would have been spent on adaptations by the council, could be used as a contribution towards a humane alternative. I would need to cover the remaining costs. It was the tail end of this type of grant that was soon to be stopped.

Following the latest occupational therapists' recommendations of the bedroom / shower / toilet ensemble, the cost of this gem of a 'tick box solution' would have shockingly cost the council much less to fulfil than the initial suggestion. The grant award had been reduced from the lift adaptations £18,000 plus, to the bargain price of £8,000 that the bedroom/shower/toilet would cost.

I used all my savings to pay for an architectural drawing to turn my backroom into a wet room and bedroom, leaving the space for the kids and me as it was. It was passed in theory but not financially. If I could find the rest of the money myself and all the works met the strict criteria set by the council, then it would be passed. I had the architect adapt the plans numerous times until it was eventually approved.

Armed with a supporting letter from the MS nurses, I wrote to various charities and other fund-raising bodies asking for help. I could then borrow the rest from family and friends. Following confirmation that I could cover the costs, the plans were approved. Next came the builders to quote for the work and I picked a chap that had done similar jobs before. He seemed extremely knowledgeable but more importantly, stupid as it might sound, was empathetic to my thirty-something-year-old-in-denial disabled self. We agreed that once the final drawing had been cleared, work could commence. I had been given a verbal go ahead but just needed an official stamp.

It was a Tuesday which meant one thing – I was off for oxygen at the MS centre. While I was there, I had a reflexology treatment (made a wonderful change to be on the receiving end!) and joined in with a group physio session. I felt good - my glasses were glowing.

I got back to the house and looked out into the garden. A huge trench had been dug. I could not believe my eyes. The next day the builders showed up, followed shortly after by a council official. As the work had commenced before I had received an official stamp, the terms of the grant had been breached. Because the work had already started, they could in theory withdraw any funding - you couldn't make it up. Here we go again, in preparation for the worst, I printed out some of my text correspondence to prove I had not asked for the work to be started. I got a copy of the MS centre sign in sheet to prove I wasn't present when the work started. Several nerve-wracking and sleepless nights later we were back on. Then it was a return to making tea for plumbers and builders but this time with my boobs away.

The MS nurses were key to keeping me "normal," although normal never sounds fun. Alongside the continence clinic, physiotherapist and occupational therapist, they referred me to another specialist clinic. This ominous sounding place focuses on each person's mobility. It turns out, when you discover you have MS, us lucky ones get to visit these specialist clinics. I went along several times over the course of six months. We tried a variety of incredible inventions to counteract, what was then explained to be, foot drop. Foot drop is massively prevalent with MS sufferers. We tried splints and elasticated equipment to pull my toes up. Each time I visited the lab, I went away with another "toy." Each of these, in turn, for various reasons failed.

Thank goodness the MS nurses aren't quitters.

One afternoon I drove out to the Gait Lab where a lovely gentleman examined how well I could stretch and bend. It turns out I could have been a ballerina with my hypermobility. The tiny tutu and constant hair buns however, would have been way too much effort. Saying that, the tutus were probably elasticated - perhaps I should change career? As it happened, my ballet dancer flexibility was probably key to keeping me out of a wheelchair. After I had been manipulated, stretched and my yoga style twists admired, I was filmed walking.

A large figure of eight had been drawn on the floor. I tentatively walked the figure of eight with my stick in hand. After observing my movement, the chap disappeared into an adjoining storage cupboard and emerged with what looked like a Walkman (remember those?) and a couple of batteries. This is where the robot version of me makes a grand entrance.

Two "nicotine patches" with wires protruding out of them were carefully positioned close to the back and the front of my naughty leg. Now the exact placements of these were key. With the Walkman in his hand, the chap pressed a button and I instantly received a sudden sharp electric shock causing my foot to flick out. Basically, I had been turned into a live circuit. This mobility maestro of a man then placed a button shaped switch into the insole of my shoe and taped it securely. This was then connected to the Walkman. Again, I was asked to walk the figure of eight. This time with my stick in one hand, the box of trickery in the other and with wires running down my leg into my boot.

I began my walk. As I put my foot down it pressed onto the pressure switch in my shoe and an electric shock travelled from the back of my leg and plummeted through my entire leg causing it to kick out. Oh my, so each step was an electric shock - oh the fun! The vast majority of us MS sufferers have dulled sensation. I didn't in this area and very much still felt this electric shock. It was clear that the circuit was working and resulting in a kick out. The objective was achieved and I headed home.

It turns out that these Walkman's or 'FES machines' by their proper name, were and probably still are, expensive bits of kit. They demanded a strong case putting forward and approval given before they could be given out. The maestro was going to send the footage and fight for my funding and he did just that.

I returned two weeks later but this time was greeted by a lady therapist. We entered the less ominous sounding Gait Lab and I took a seat. The lady therapist went into the same adjoining storage room and returned with a Walkman of my very own. She attached the patches to my leg and turned it on. The positioning didn't seem to come together as readily this time and my foot didn't kick out as profoundly.

The sharp pain was still there however. Where was the Maestro? I was instructed to take it home and play about with it until the positioning seemed right and got the desired effect. She personally couldn't see much difference. "That's because you've put it in the wrong place," I thought to myself.

The next day I got myself all circuited up and my goodness it was painful. I went to the local park, switched it on and then took my first step. The electric charge rushed through me as soon as my boot hit the ground. I stopped dead in my stride and balanced on one leg in what I like to call my flamingo pose. I took a deep breath and then took another step, the shock ran through me again. Perhaps I really didn't need to be at the park. I turned around and took another step to be greeted with the familiar electric surge. By this point, my eyes had filled with tears. I took another step, slightly biting my lip. I would get used to it, surely. I took a deep breath in and stepped towards the car, with my nostrils flared, my lips quivering and a single tear ran down my cheek. I was tougher than this – wasn't I? I promised myself that I'd try again tomorrow before I headed home feeling deflated.

The next day I had my breakfast in the morning, then sat staring at my boot and the wired nicotine patches. "Do you want to walk or not," I asked myself. My mantra, whilst injecting myself, was "I am walking, I'm not going to need a wheelchair." While chanting the words I plunged a needle into my own leg. That was just once on alternate days before it became a weekly occasion. Currently, I went into the hospital for a two-hour infusion every month, which is why an electric shock with every step seemed a bit cruel. "Do you want to walk or not," I said crossly to myself again. I had dealt with pain so what the hell was wrong with me? Maybe I could take pain killers if I wanted to go anywhere. Now I was just being ridiculous. I acknowledged that I would set it up tomorrow instead - after all, I had to be at school for the pick-up in a few hours.

I was feeling a bit hard done by. I've never actually asked the question, that is expected on diagnosis; "Why me?"

A very kind man (referring to my holistic treatments) said to me "your healing ability will help you. Some people like yourself, seem to be chosen to experience many worldly problems, so they can understand the hardships of others. Use your god given healing ability to help yourself."

Now this makes me sound like I'm some sort of incredible being. I am extremely honoured that this lovely gentleman put me in such a kind light but I would say that I'm just very stubborn. In my short-ish life so far, I've had a few stumbling blocks - I've just always managed to turn them into stepping stones but that's another tale.

I wasn't on top form at the minute, my glasses needed polishing - step forth number 9! With her arm and folded up stick, we headed off into town for drinks. We were initially confronted by a doorman who was convinced that I was obviously already too drunk to enter the premises. My breath grew heavy and smiles started to fall, here we go again…

"She's fine. I know her," a female bouncer called out who was also working on the doors.

The words were said just before I had to reach into my bag and pull out my stick by way of ID to prove myself. I clung onto number 9 so I didn't fall and because I was way too stubborn to show that I needed help. We sat down at a table and number 9 went to fetch pitchers of BOGOF cocktails. In the past, we'd discovered that as I drank alcohol, my walking improved. Perhaps it was something to do with the brain transmissions that make most people start stumbling straightened me up? All I had to do was become an alcoholic. There were several issues with this a) the boy, b) the little lady, c) I had to drive to get from anywhere to anywhere.

Number 9 placed two jugs of our favourite tipples on our table. As she did so, familiar and unfamiliar faces arrived. When people discover you are single they immediately try to set you up with someone. I hadn't been single for a very long time and planned to stay single for a very long time. I had to concentrate on my beautiful little people and work out how to make my legs work.

"This is the Plumber and the Yorkshire man - they're both single." One of the group proclaimed by way of introduction.

"I'm not surprised," I answered rudely.

I was not interested in anyone at all, I had more important issues on my plate. The two men and two other ladies from the group returning from the bar sat down with me and number 9. The Yorkshire man made a comment about the potent but murky looking drink sat in front of me. I had a very long, uninteresting conversation with the uninteresting man, who was equally as disinterested in me as I was in him. The uninteresting man had to leave as he had to go to his uninteresting job in the morning.

I love music and so, minus the uninteresting man, we all went to the bar directly opposite, which had loud music blaring from behind its doors. Several strangers offered me drinks and even to buy me dinner. I'm not sure if as you become a single person, your relationship status becomes glaringly obvious. Maybe I had a radar alerting every available man in the nearby vicinity? It certainly wasn't because I was very approachable, in fact, I'm ashamed to say quite the opposite. For what I hope was the first and last time in my life, I was terribly dismissive and abrupt to any male who even glanced my way. The matchmaking saga continued as different people in our group kept handing me the uninteresting man's details. I was not interested however and nor was he.

Over in the music filled bar, if my leg made me stumble, I just turned it into a dance move. The more drinks I had, the less I stumbled and the more other people did - ironic really. Number 9 and I danced the night away. My glasses were gleaming beautifully. Even if I did have a wonky leg, I was still attractive, or perhaps that was because everyone had beer goggles on. Previously, whenever we went out, I'd borrowed a ring from number 9 to make it look as if I was married, not that it seemed to make a huge difference to the patrolling male species. I had always been desperate to be married, in order to complete my perfect family. Now, I was starting to realise that the universe / god / fate, sometimes changes your path. A path that previously included 2.4 smiling children, the picket fence and the perfect, doting and loving husband.

Later that week, I messaged the uninteresting man, after all, I hadn't got anything more interesting to do and the kids were busy playing. Myself and the equally uninterested Yorkshire man, continued to send many uninteresting messages to one another in the hours, days and weeks to follow.

10

The Monster Gets Some Tears

The adaptations to the house were finished the week before Christmas making it the perfect gift. This had however delayed putting up the decorations by around three weeks. As soon as the last work was completed and I'd waved goodbye to the last builder, I rushed – well, in a limpy "one leg at a time" fashion - up the stairs to get the decorations out. The panic leg lifting was to be a thing of the past. I breathed a huge sigh of relief - I now had a downstairs wet room with a folding seat so I could sit and shower, as opposed to the council proposal of a cubicle to shit and shower. I now had a downstairs bedroom too, not my original plan but it would make life much easier. My boy and my little lady were getting nearly as excited about Christmas as me. I had bought festive bits and pieces throughout the year, as the thought of buying everything in one go was horrendous. Turns out, they had more than ever with the little bargains I'd picked up throughout the year, in my single-parent-panicked-thoughts about the kids not having a full Christmas. I wouldn't be spending all of Christmas with the kids but I smiled to myself knowing that despite this, it would be a great Christmas.

We were running late to take the little lady to school. The electric nicotine patches took too long to put on in the correct position I told myself which excused me from putting them on - no shocks today. I drove to the school and pulled right up to my allocated parking space. Her classroom was straight across the playground, a mere stone's throw. I reached over for my stick and got out of the car. She had already got out of the car with her packed lunch in hand and her rucksack (nearly the same size as her) on her back. I took one step then did the classic and fell over nothing. The little lady screamed out "Mummy!" as I smashed my face on the floor. Having the stick in my hand meant I hadn't been able to put my hands out in front of me I thought, trying to rationalise why I fell. I was cross, I'd had the luxury of a seated shower this morning, I hadn't needed to tackle any stairs so my legs shouldn't be failing me. My little lady was crying over me but with all of my might, I stood up quickly and said "I'm fine, I'm fine," with an over the top fake smile plastered on my face. I brushed my hands together to clear them of the bits of car park. My little girl ran and picked up my flyaway stick and we walked over to her classroom. I couldn't allow this to happen - next time, I would just have to grit my teeth with every step and use the cursed FES machine. I should really feel grateful that I could still feel my legs but my word it was painful.

Both kids were going to stay with their father that night. I was off to a friend's 40th birthday party and the uninteresting Yorkshire man was accompanying me. Number 9 was there along with many mutual friends and extended friendship groups. As I stood at the bar to get some drinks, one of the girls (a friend of a friend) came up beside me. Her sister had Multiple Sclerosis and had just had treatment that was "amazing" and had apparently done wonders for her. She had been using a wheelchair and was now walking everywhere. She begged me to go along to a presentation about the treatment that her sister was involved in the following week. She advised that I could at least go and ask questions. I had been dealing with this monster for twelve years and it wasn't about to go anywhere anytime soon. I was still having a monthly infusion, had stabbed myself for years and after examining my diet in an attempt to help my symptoms, I was now gluten and dairy-free. I didn't think a talk would be of any use. It does get tiresome when everyone has a cure for something you've been dealing with for longer than a decade. She was persistent though and I had nothing else to do. What on earth did adults do when they were childless?

The meeting place was just round the corner from where I lived, so was only a two-minute drive. The uninteresting Yorkshire man offered to come with me. I still hated driving so I took him up on the offer. As we parked up I saw a woman walking in a similar drunken slide fashion to myself, also with a stick in her hand. It was a Sunday and the main front entrance was locked, so she and her 'partner' were similarly looking for the way in. The man with her turned to both of us "wait here and I'll go see if the entrance is round the back."

He sprinted off, in the Yorkshireman's words "like a whippet." He returned to where we were stood and by this point we had introduced ourselves.

"It's round here."

The door opened into a large hall. Rows of chairs had been set out at the front of a stage where the presentation was to be made. They were sparsely filled with people, mostly older than me. I noticed some wheelchairs and every other seat had a walking stick placed neatly against the chair in front or lay on the polished hardwood floor beside them.

The presentation slides were projected onto the huge screen and the sound was checked. Various people in the room shuffled microphones and papers. It all looked terribly corporate but there were biscuits and tea and coffee available and I had my handy flask of soya milk. The uninteresting Yorkshire man went and got me a cuppa. Weirdly, he didn't have hot drinks. A Yorkshire man who doesn't drink tea, now that is interesting.

"HSCT" popped up on the screen along with what appeared to be this organisation's name, it had started. One by one enthusiastic, happy looking people stood on the stage and spoke about their experiences of Stem Cell Treatment for MS. I'd previously asked a medical professional I'll call "X" about this crazy treatment after I'd seen it featured on a TV documentary; apparently, fifty per cent of those that had the treatment had gotten even worse or had died. I was told this by someone in the know. I remember thinking I'd have to be on death's door to even bother looking into it. My kids were better off with me around even if it was in a wheelchair but I was here so I may as well listen. The group had nothing but positive attributes and testimonies about the Stem Cell Treatment. They spoke of people's symptoms improving and getting a new lease of life. A lady with bright red hair ran across the room to get the microphone, then proceeded to tell us how she had been in a wheelchair less than a year ago. Hmmm, was I expected to believe in this miracle cure? If this was real, then why wasn't everyone having it? Why would I and thousands of others like me be needlessly self-harming with needles? It turned out that bright red-haired woman was the sister of the person from the bar I was here to have a chat with.

As it happens, the previously encountered entrance finding whippet had also had the treatment. Others from the group continued to share their miraculous stories. They proceeded to show videos of hospitals in London, Mexico and Russia that could offer the treatment. There were clips of specialist doctors from the respective clinics. Lots of the speakers came off as highly intelligent and seemed to be able to spiel off facts and figures beautifully without any hitches.

A tiny man, with a large grin wearing a white coat, appeared on screen and began talking about his family all over the world. He spoke, what sounded to me, about hippy love and science going hand in hand. He was a funny little man but if I was ever going to be stupid enough to try something like this, I'd want that hippy scientist to do it and in Russia. Ha - as if I'd ever go to Russia, big scary cold place, I smirked to myself. The success rates around HSCT (Stem Cell treatment) were vastly different from what I'd previously been told. As the presentation came to an end, the equally hobble-y lady from the car park grabbed my hand and said to me "You can do it, I'm going in February" and gave me a squeeze.

What? No, I was just killing some time without the kids.

Shortly after we moved into our new house, we'd had a salon built in the back garden. It was a converted outbuilding that was done so that I could carry on working. I was still happily working and had become an expert in hiding my Achilles heel - the MS. I always ensured that I was in my room before my client and had everything ready. I had a hiding place for my stick inside the room and a wooden stick in the bush outside the entrance just in case I needed to rush out for anything. Most people were either too relaxed to notice or in hindsight, perhaps felt rude asking. There were times when I found it tough. Sometimes, I would lose my balance and stumble, sometimes it was just a struggle to move. I used various excuses at the beginning; cramp, I'd fallen (this wasn't a lie, I was always falling) but it was starting to become difficult to hide my leg that dragged. I wanted people to focus on themselves and not take pity on this poor sick woman. I didn't want pity – I really didn't want pity. I loved my job and I loved helping people.

My routine annual neurologist meeting was booked in. I took the little lady to school, then I did a full body massage on a client before driving to the hospital. I arrived at my usual blue badge parking space – it had gone! Panic set in. I drove around the car park, nothing. I went to the next car park but that was too far to walk. I looked at the clock on the car radio, I was going to be late and it had started raining - I had to hurry up. I had my walking poles in the boot of the car so I got them out and pretty much dragged myself for what seemed like miles to the entrance. I went inside, soaking wet - I looked like a drowned rat. I found the nearest loo. I was very late and saturated but not making it to the toilet was not going to be added to my list.

Using my poles almost like crutches now, I made it to the clinic's reception desk. I stated my name as I peered through the misty lenses of my less than rose-tinted glasses. I was asked to take a seat. I did so and cleaned the lenses as I waited. It took quite a while but a doctor I wasn't familiar with, beckoned me into his room. I dragged my exhausted self over. The school run, a full body massage, a distant car parking spot, the wind and the rain had taken its toll today. I sat and smiled, admittedly breathing heavily with nervous exhaustion. He scrolled through my records on the screen in front of him and cited medical facts about me.

"You were diagnosed in 2007, you've been on two DMTs" (Disease Modifying Treatments, for those of you blessed with not knowing). I nodded.

"Now on Tysabri but slowly progressing and getting worse."

At that point, my eyes glazed slightly, it wasn't the condensation on my glasses unfortunately. The exact wording of what was said escapes me, but it seemed to go along the lines of, "Tysabri isn't working. There's nothing else the NHS can do for you. You'll inevitably be in a wheelchair before long

I'm sorry."

Hang on – what about the meeting? The miracle cure?

"What about Stem Cell Treatment?" I blurted out in desperation.

He explained that I was too far gone and it wouldn't work for me. No, no I wasn't going to be dismissed, I was absolutely not giving up that easily. I was insistent that he refer me to the London hospital that offered the treatment. After an initial dismissal due to it being pointless, my referral request was noted.

I have no idea how I dragged my deflated body back to my car but the second I collapsed onto the seat, I burst into tears. I rang the Yorkshire man and just wept. This was the first time in years that the monster had stolen so many tears from my eyes. Once home, I rang the MS nurses and left messages, should I be stopping treatment now? Had he referred me yet?

I contacted the red-haired lady from the meeting and got contact details for the London hospitals she'd been to. She set the stage and virtually held my hand and supported me in my "I'm not a quitter" plight. I arranged a private consultation with a senior London Neurologist who had greater expertise and knowledge of the treatment. He was fantastic - I guess you get what you pay for. He told me about several treatments that were possibilities, including one that speeded up the brain signals to the body's response. I asked him about Stem Cell Treatment.

"To get it on the NHS you would need to have active lesions." he explained.

He said that he would see if he could see any on the scans that we would be forwarding after my consultation. He told me he had heard positive reports from clinics in Mexico and Russia but obviously that would need paying for privately.

A couple of months later, I received a letter to tell me that the hospital I'd been referred to didn't offer Stem Cell Treatment for MS. Unbelievably, I'd been referred to the wrong hospital. Was this an accident or an act of sabotage (insert menacing grin)? I rang the MS nurses the same day and they chased the referral. I was eventually passed over to the correct hospital but ultimately received the highly frustrating response that I was not eligible.

I continued to go for my monthly infusions. The nurses had become friends, counsellors and supporters too. I'd been going for two hours, every twenty-eight days, for six years without fail, so these nurses probably knew me better than many of my friends. Over the next few days, I exchanged many messages with my red-haired miracle lady. She answered everything I wanted to know without exception. I was fired up. I wanted to see that scientific hippy in Russia! The Yorkshire man was finding this all terribly interesting.

11

Life without the glasses

Iwas definitely going for it. 'A wheelchair by Christmas'- I don't think so! I got my laptop out and started searching for the Russian hospital that was going to stop my MS progression and allow me to stick two fingers up as part of the deal. Firstly, the application.

I needed medical records which was not as easy as I'd anticipated. After a few fruitless and blatant conversations with receptionists and call handlers, I was eventually pointed in the direction of the internet. Due to the ever changing laws on accessing personal information, applying for your full medical records was actually quite straightforward. Karma was clearly still helping me out. It took about a month for the records to arrive but when they did, I had a mountain of dates, scans and X-rays to plough through. It took me on a huge nostalgic trip of accidents and incidents - really cool to see. I pretended to myself that I knew what the medical jargon meant while quickly scanning through, mostly guessing according to the corresponding dates. Any doctor or Accident and Emergency visit was detailed in clinical babble and reported in shorthand note form.

In hindsight, looking through the reasons for going to the doctors in the first place - the signs were all there - it all fitted together like a puzzle. The amount of bumph was huge. I was thankful that I wasn't a hypochondriac and only used the doctors as a last resort. I favoured random plants, herbs or concoctions using essential oils and natural ingredients to treat ailments.

I went back to the online application filling in incident dates, diagnoses, medications and relapses. After several nights with little sleep, the detailed email was sent. Within days I received a reply. The smiley Russian doctor had reviewed my case and it was decided that I was a suitable candidate for the treatment. This put a ginormous grin on my face. Despite what I'd previously been told there was something more that could be done and I was hell bent on doing it!

Furthermore, the e-mail went on to say they'd had a cancellation and could get me in for treatment in three months. It sounded great but they required the full payment upfront, which was thousands and thousands; enough for a two bed house (in a less desirable area admittedly). It was an unimaginable amount of money - I was a single mum of two. I had managed to blag my way through life so far and keep two little beings fed, not to mention the rescued cats, chickens, dogs, rabbits, chinchilla, guinea pigs and sea monkeys. A smile, good karma and crossed fingers can take you far. I was determined that I would have the money within a year. I had no idea how yet but I would – that much I was certain about. I politely replied asking them to defer the place. I messaged the red-haired miracle regularly with my ideas and thoughts for raising money. She shared how she had similarly raised funds and pretty much coached me from start to finish.

The first thing to do was to set up a fundraising page. A few brief enquiries and calls for advice later and I'd chosen a personal fundraising page to use. Again, it was quite straightforward and it was at this point the catchphrase emerged; "Kezia Kicks Back." To run alongside this, I had a Facebook page set up and run by a friend who turns out had a flair for raffles. The world of Twitter was smothered with images, videos and links all under the banner of "Kezia Kicks Back." I shared ideas for fundraising events in my close circles of friends. I'm lucky in that I have a few circles of friends, all with very different quirks and sparkles. The Bakewell Tarts (house mates from Uni) told me to record my day to day happenings. It was to provide a very real fly on the wall insight into the world of an MS sufferer. This would be okay, I'd video me getting ready for work, doing house stuff, playing with kids or while sitting in the garden. That wasn't the idea apparently and this would in fact, be the hardest thing in the world for me.

I recorded the reality 'behind the rose-tints' and everything I'd spent years hiding from everyone around me, I put on film. The frustration, the tears, the anger and bruises from trips over nothing were out for the world to see and comment on if they chose to. If I was going to go to the scariest and coldest place in the world to meet the hippy scientist, I had to "come out." I started filming hospital visits, my infusions and all the things I had hidden for more than ten years. They were now going to be on a platter for all to see in broad daylight. The world would see behind my rose-tinted glasses. I pinched myself

- on film was everything I'd spent years hiding from others and even more frighteningly, myself. It had taken up a lot of energy doing so.

I was so busy proving that "I was fine" and could cope just as well as everyone else, that I'd fooled myself in the process. I had put my fingers in my ears, buried my head in the sand and had gone "la, la, la." These video snippets were a harsh slap in the face to me and involved me having to remove my rose-tinted glasses; now that was frightening but the Yorkshire man held my glasses and wiped them when they were misty.

The Just Giving fundraiser website was great. The first lot of donations were from people I hadn't seen since primary school. Just a little while ago, the donations kept coming from family, friends, acquaintances and complete strangers. It was quite staggering.

It was at this point my boy turned to me and remarked, "there's obviously something in this karma stuff you go on about."

After discussing various events that had successfully worked for her, the red haired miracle and I decided to host a pamper day; the first fundraiser. My young mum, Patrick and a few friends all stepped up. We even managed to rope the kids in to help. The living room was transformed into our pamper suite. The red haired one was doing nails and I offered head and hand massages. In the kitchen was a large table completely covered with tombola prizes. Patrick ran this and was on great form in showman mode and aced at getting people to part with their pennies. Young Mum was selling various craft items while encouraging people to guess the name of a large teddy bear. A friend was painting little people's faces and of course there was the obligatory and hugely popular cake stall. Delicious! Between clients, the red haired miracle was amazing people with stories of how she'd gone from wheelchair to walking after having the treatment. Everyone seemed astounded, myself included.

After we'd gained our diplomas in Holistics, my fellow 20 percenter and I had the pleasure of working in our first salon alongside two beautiful ladies. This trio had taken upon themselves to arrange another fundraiser between them. This time it was to be a party, with all eyes very much on me. It was, I thought, possibly the most attention I would ever have. A wonderful thing for a theatre student. Trust me.

The trio had everyone send in a song request that reminded them in some way of me. These and a list of my own song choices were made into what was probably the best playlist ever. My 20 percenter had made the most amazing cake with butterflies and my name on it! The butterflies were there in representation of my business, Kelebek (Turkish for butterfly).

In my own words, "the emerging butterfly is not the creation of something stunning but the unveiling of something beautiful, that was there all along."

There was a Kezia-themed quiz which included a picture round of yours truly, 'Kezia Kicks Back' cocktails and the main event - the charity auction to which many people had generously donated items and services. The girls raised loads of cash, smiles, MS awareness and shared marvellous memories. Family, friends, clients, (and friends of) all came to the party fundraiser. The efforts the girls went to made me feel so deeply loved and I realised how important I was to them and them to me.

Patrick really took to the fundraising. Being a fellow thespian himself, shouting from the roof tops for cash and asking for help from anyone who'd listen came naturally. He had landed a set on community radio and one of the fellow DJs answered his plea and offered to host a fundraiser for me. This was set to be completely different and unexpected; Fundraiser 3: The Spiritualists. This lovely group were going to offer spiritual readings and healing throughout the day, alongside other stalls offering Henna tattoos, crystals, handmade jewellery and all manner of rose-tinted equipment (right up my street). As I hobbled into the hall of strangers, I felt a warmth that was hard to explain. I took a seat on one of the brown plastic chairs. Just as I did, a beautiful delicate little lady approached me with some money scrunched in her hand. She handed it to me and then scuttled away. She came straight back, arms wide-spread displaying a huge multi-coloured hand crocheted blanket.

"I made this for you and I've covered it in Reiki. I thought you would like it in many colours." She was correct.

This huge hall of strangers coming together, to raise money so I could keep living my wonderful life on my own two feet, was a reinforcement of the kindness of these people.

A completely different day was arranged by the kid's grandad. He is a huge film fan so it was fitting that he arranged an outside screening, in one of - what I would refer to as - my happy places. This Eco hotspot had everything; vegan food (and cakes) and promoted all things green. I'd taken the little man when he was small and then the little lady. My little man had proudly returned home brandishing a cardboard sword and recycled plastic drum with accompanying beater. The young lady and I made a fairy door and fairy wings after we had hunted fairies and ate cake.

For two months leading up to the screening, the whole family became ticket touts, going no-where without a wad just in case. The little lady's school promoted the event through newsletters, we advertised it on the social media pages and basically sold to anyone who showed the slightest interest. It was an unbelievably difficult job and I now have full respect for those that do it for a living. As the day of the screening drew closer, the weather was not playing nicely. It was difficult enough to get people to pay for something in advance but the rain forecasted was making it even harder. We persevered.

The day came and my trusted face painter was sat with me, next to the obligatory raffle in a yurt. As people began to arrive, the huge screen had gone up with rows of chairs and space for blankets. The mobile bar was set up and ready but then came the rain. The eco staff were incredible. They had set up an inside screen for little ones to see the show before bedtime and they now brought our outdoor evening screening inside too. Any face painted people began to resemble an obscure Picasso painting. I'm sure we lost some paying customers because of the weather but family, friends and the Yorkshire man's gang helped to raise a chunk of cash and the perseverance of everyone made the whole day a lot of fun.

The next few months were a non-stop frenzy of activity. Every week there would be a different fundraising event of some sort and hosted by friends, family and acquaintances. We had garden parties held by close friends and a wildcard played by some friends of my Dad's from back in the day. They'd seen that I was raising funds and kindly offered to arrange a cheese and wine night and auction. This was a massive bolt out of the blue given that my dad had died thirteen years before.

My redhead miracle had told me about a large local restaurant that gave a cut of their buffet takings to any pre-arranged charity nights. We pretty much filled the place, complete with a fantastic and uplifting atmosphere for the evening.

Some events went a lot better than others but at the end of the day, they were all for a common cause. The treatment was an unbelievable amount of money but what price do you put on your quality of life? I also had to factor in flights, visas, hotels and consider physio and after treatment too.

I lay belly down on the bed with my head resting on cupped hands thinking about the things that I needed for Russia. The kids were milling about, the boy with his head in the fridge sniffing out any unhealthy calorie laden food and the girl pushing two of her many children in a pushchair. Mum and Patrick were chatting to the Yorkshire man in the kitchen about the arrangements once we were back from Russia.

Even though Moscow was still a way off, there was almost a sense of urgency in the air whenever the subject arose. Although no one said it, the excitement, apprehension and anticipation was clearly felt and shared by everyone. There was a cool rush of air, as if someone had opened the front door. One of my musketeers walked into my room. My pub crawl musketeer had an envelope in her hand. For reasons to be mentioned at a later point, I remember what happened in great detail. She looked uneasy but smiled, perhaps the ambience was apparent.

"My mum had one of her open gardens. I made and sold cakes to put towards your treatment. It's not much but hope it helps."

"Thank you so much monkey, it will definitely

and tell your mum thank you too. We need to make sure we have a catch up when I'm back from Russia." I pulled an exaggerated scared face.

She nodded, "Looks like you've got your hands full, I just wanted to nip in before you go."

Then, she rushed off. There were also some astounding and very generous donations from my family.

I hadn't read much about the intricacies of the procedure but I knew it wasn't going to be a barrel of laughs. I was going to be leaving my babies in England and heading to Russia to have chemo. Although this seemed insane, I had run out of choices and I was not going to let this monster, MS, take me away from my kids.

The Yorkshire man, the two kids and I went away for a short break in the UK. I wanted them to have memories of me smiling and with hair (as unbelievably vain as it sounds). I had huge thick curls and would be returning home to them shockingly bald and probably pretty ill. The Yorkshire man persuaded me to hire an electric scooter while we were away. This went against every single rule I had committed myself to and those familiar words echoed in my head

"Don't be too stubborn to not use a wheelchair, but remember that once you get in, it's near impossible to get out."

It hurt when we ordered it but it was so worth it. My boy, now a teenager, begged to take turns. For the first time, since before he was in double digits and never for the little lady, they both had to run to keep up with me. Incredible!

12

The Warriors and
Leopard Print Pants

Russia is notoriously difficult to enter. As I discovered, on top of a very in depth and expensive visa application, you also have to have an invite into the country. Everything had to be approved, signed and countersigned.

The application for a visa was harder than my dissertation. Apart from usual basic questions such as the duration and purpose of the visit, where we were staying, with whom, where we'd be going and how much we'd be spending, the forms demanded a lot more information. It was tiring to look at but I charged ahead fuelled by my vision of a better quality life. The details required included; the full names, dates of birth, addresses, occupation, full passport details, dates and all trips abroad for not only myself over the last ten years but most of it also applied for my parents and children too. Pretty much everything that could have been asked, was asked, including when and where my father had passed away. Once this was complete, I'd have to find my way to the Russian application centre in London for fingerprints to be taken.

The Yorkshire man accompanied me to the Russian visa centre. Tackling transport in London, when your legs don't do what they're told is horrendous. I immediately ruled out the underground. We took a National Express coach to London, then hailed down a smiley faced hackney cab driver. As expected, he knew exactly where it was and the quickest route to get there. He weaved his way through the backstreets of London, zoomed down bus lanes and got me within a stone's throw of the entrance. Perfect.

Armed with a rucksack of important documentation and a bank card, we stepped into the Visa Application Centre. The whole thing was surprisingly straightforward and painless with hardly any waiting around. Despite the dauntingly stern faces of the office staff, a few hours later and minus a large amount of cash, we were heading back home.

The all-inclusive trip to Russia included my breakfast, brunch, lunch, dinner, supper and snacks in a luxury five-star hospital in the centre of Moscow. All this for the bargain sum of around £40,000 give or take allowing for the exchange rate and handling fees. So how on earth was I going to send this sort of money to Russia? This wasn't exactly the same as putting a gift voucher in a birthday card. Step forward the "YOU CAN DO IT" lady from the initial presentation. She'd been for the same treatment in Moscow months before and she put me on the right track, giving me the details of a company who dealt with this type of transaction. First of all, I had to explain to my bank what would be happening so not to raise any concerns. Large sums of money leaving one's bank account to be transferred to another country is likely to be marked with red flags. Money was already coming in from all over the world via the fundraising. Trust me, I realised how lucky I was but at the same time, I saw how crazy it must seem. A hard-core medical procedure in Russia had never been on my to-do-list, mind you, neither was MS.

If someone were to tell me they were having treatment abroad, I'd imagine glamorous and wannabe models having boob jobs, liposuction or their noses sculpted at a more attractive price ticket than in the UK. On the other end of the spectrum was euthanasia. This treatment didn't fit into my massively stereotypical view either. Many people, both friends and family, got in contact. "You realise how dangerous this treatment is?" "This could actually kill you?" and "the chemo is stronger than they give to cancer patients," were some of the most common remarks.

I just put on my rose-tinted glasses and smiled, after all, I could blag my way through anything. Admittedly, I hadn't actually done much research into the medical side. I'd focused on fundraising so that my happy hippy doctor could focus on that aspect. My every day focus, was looking after my little people, remaining standing and raising cash so I could keep doing both of those.

Next to organise were the flights and a hotel - my goodness there were lots of hidden extras I had not even thought about. These were terribly pricey extras but necessary for the end goal - keeping my wonderful life. I had a beautiful home and garden, with many regular bird and animal visitors. I had a fabulous job, with amazing clients and I was mum to two scrumptious growing big little people. Like the advert says "what money can't buy…is priceless."

My hospital admission was arranged. I had a Russian visa in my passport and the invite into the country was sorted. Economy flights for my departure were booked and I had premium economy flights booked for on the journey back. I was told it was safer than regular economy seating, less kids on board I guess. As a mother, I am allowed to say the following; kids are extremely germ ridden creatures best to be avoided, especially after your immune system has been zapped by chemo.

Taxis were scheduled, bags were packed with headscarves, pyjamas and tea bags. My favourite tea was an essential. Having joined an online group for those who'd been for the treatment and those who were going to be in the hospital at the same time as me, I'd been warned that I needed flavourings such as cinnamon, salt and pepper. This group would later be my lifeline.

My young mum, my little people and myself, were armed with tablets, ready for video calls, courtesy of the Yorkshire man. I had Audible in place so I could be read to and do some research for my work. Is it still counted as work if it's your hobby and passion?

The day came. Everything had been packed,

unpacked, checked and checked again and my luggage was lined up perfectly at the front door. The taxi was booked for perhaps a little too early but there was no way I was missing that flight to Russia. I still couldn't believe I was going. My son had downloaded an app so I could learn Russian; if there was a woman drinking milk on the Metro I would be able to tell her where her jumper was and ask for bread. What else could I possibly need to know?

The taxi arrived and I hobbled towards it. The driver opened the boot, walked towards me and took one of the cases. Using a stick automatically ensures that you do not carry your own luggage. The Yorkshire man was going to accompany me. The plan was for him to drop me off, return to England and then he would go back to Russia to collect me afterwards. I wonder if the insanity of dropping off this wonky lady to a hospital in Moscow, to have chemo, would make his year a bit more interesting. It was certainly out of my comfort zone, a trip to Russia, never mind the reason I was going.

I was going to fly to a top hospital in another country, have chemo, lose all of my hair, then fly back. As mad as it sounded, I had done no real research into the science of the procedure. I instead focused on the most important parts. Maybe somewhere along the way, I may have been more scared if I had explored it in more detail and perhaps it was better not to know? I had my rose-tinted glasses to maintain after all.

Losing my huge thick brown mop of curls as a sacrifice for not ending up in a wheelchair seemed like a fair swap. I did love my shaggy mane though. I could leave it au naturel, or quickly tie it up in a pony out of the way. Everyone else of my gender it seemed, spent a fortune on dyes, hair-dressers and potions - mine was lazy hair. I'd been told it might come back completely different, wow that was exciting - I could come back as a blonde or with poker straight locks. I'd had DIY shades of red, orange, black and blonde highlights but to straighten my curls would take a professional and many hours of labour.

We arrived at the airport and we checked in mega early, dropped off our luggage and went to sit in one of the cafes. It was in fact, all very unremarkable and straightforward. I did hope the rest of this insanity would be along the same ilk but I had a strong inkling it may not be.

The flight was a lot shorter than I'd expected. Russia, I still couldn't believe it. The language alone sounded like nothing I'd ever heard. Surely it would be a twenty-four-hour flight? Turns out it was about four. We stepped off the plane and into the airport to be greeted with signs written in dashes and dots, that didn't even appear to be like words. The devoted Yorkshire man carried our bags. His bag was small, a tenth of the size of mine. His return flight was booked for five days later, leaving enough time to get me settled into the hospital. Once in Arrivals, there were people waiting holding up cardboard signs with names on. I spotted my name but mine stood out as it was on an iPad - clearly a sign I was paying big money! The gentleman introduced himself, took the bags and amazingly managed to rush us through immigration, passport control and settled us into his taxi. He told us via Google Translate how the Russian government had made tunnels under the roads, so wildlife could move freely without being squished. Perhaps the Russians weren't as cut-throat as they appear on films.

We had booked a hotel for a couple of days before I started being tested at the hospital. I had been quite blasé about the testing, as I had with every aspect of the treatment. After the flight I wanted to just chill. I posted on the group forum that I had arrived and we arranged to meet some of the other patients and their plus ones. The next day we all had dinner together at a restaurant in a nearby hotel. They all seemed remarkably positive and excited. No negativity could be sniffed out whatsoever. Rose-tinted glasses were worn by the lot of them. They were warriors not victims. The group were from all over the UK, Holland, Norway, Australia and New Zealand too. It became more and more obvious as the time went by in the Russian hospital, that we were all similar characters. I am yet to decide if it's that we are all absolutely bonkers or born fighters, I'm hoping it's the latter. We all put a finger up to MS and carried some kind of "fuck it bucket."

I love seafood and as I looked through the Italian menu I found myself drawn to my favourite, Pasta Marinara. As I discussed my potential dinner choice I felt a few concerned eyes upon me. Across the table a fellow patient to be was also perusing the menu, apparently drawn towards ordering a steak. He also received looks of concern, mainly from his wife. I wanted the fish, I couldn't have the fish. Similarly, he fancied a steak, his wife said he couldn't have the steak. We had made it all the way to Russia and paid up front, not to mention an epic battle with the Visa applications, so now I was about to risk food poisoning for a Marinara? Alright, I got it. I frowned inwardly like a spoilt child and ordered a

Margherita; that's pizza – not the famous cocktail! My inner child pulled a hugely dramatic yawn face.

I had been informed that the process began with testing. If we were going to do the beep test I wanted to call number 9 to back up my story. Nope, turns out that these tests were MRI's, X-rays and blood tests. No problems to be seen here, I'd had billions of scans. Apart from my exorcist introduction to the scanner, I was the MRI queen. I wasn't fazed at all by being in the enclosed tunnel of the machine, I just meditated. You may as well make good use of the time.

Day one of testing arrived. The Yorkshire man and I were to be picked up from outside the hotel by a driver from the clinic. A rather large and swanky black car pulled up. The driver came out, dressed as you would expect a chauffeur to be and took my cases. The hospital grounds were beautiful with trees planted everywhere. The air was warm and there was not a fur hat in sight. I went to the office of the hippy scientist. He was a tiny smiley man, whose hair didn't resemble Einstein's at all. He was very welcoming and informative, although I have to be honest, I plastered a smile on my face then completely zoned out. I blame the brain fog, the perfect excuse. In truth, it was probably the realisation of what I was actually about to do. I was escorted to a teeny room with all the basic facilities, it seemed pleasant enough.

It wasn't long before the door was knocked and a chap with a wheelchair in tow beckoned me. I sat in the wheelchair, trusting of me I know but surely when in hospital you just do what you're told. Well mostly, thinking back to most definitely not doing as I was told about the cyst when I was pregnant with the little lady.

First came the expected MRI for which I was told to undress, no problems there. A short journey down the corridor and I was then told to sit in a chair which was then raised. Being just five foot one and a smidge, it wasn't long before I was sat in mid-air, legs dangling, in t-shirt and pants with a heavy hairdresser style bib over my shoulders. I was told to open my mouth, now this was really bloody weird. A scanning machine like something from Star Wars pointed at me. Then came the voice of a Russian Alanis Morrisette assertively directing me,

"Tilt your head back and relax your shoulders. Open your mouth wider."

So surreal. This, I assumed was a one-off experience and I later found out from another patient that it was a sinus x-ray. I planned to go back to the hotel but testing would commence again early in the morning, so I was advised to stay at the clinic. The poor Yorkshire man headed back to the hotel. He would have to fend Moscow solo and make his way back to the hospital tomorrow. He would not be able to tell any milk drinking ladies the sweater wasn't his.

I was wheeled back to my room. There were two specimen pots. One was clearly for a urine sample - those were common in my world - the second was much larger. Then I realised, that one was for my poop and I immediately became constipated. This may however have been due to the sudden introduction of dairy and wheat back into my diet. I didn't want to cause a fuss though, these people catered for MSer's all day long. They knew their stuff.

It wasn't the next morning that testing continued, it was in fact that evening. This time it was a Russian nurse that arrived at my door with a wheelchair. I obediently jumped in and we whizzed off, only stopping to gather another nurse who was pushing an occupied wheelchair. The ladies moved swiftly through the corridors and into the lifts down to the depths of the hospital. We suddenly stopped outside a door. My dark haired, blue-eyed wheelchair driving lady said in a very sharp Russian accent "you go in and remove the clothes."

I could make out a shadow in the corner of the room...and I thought the sinus X-ray was weird? There was a hospital bed in the middle of the room. The wheelchair chauffeur put her hands out and mimicked taking something off her shoulder. I stripped down until I was just stood in my under-wear. She pointed at my bra "off, then lay up there" in an equally stern manner.

I did as I was told and she muttered something else. I had no idea what it was but I know milk or sweaters weren't mentioned and then she left the room. The shadow in the corner turned into a sil-houette and then into a man, a very young man. He looked anywhere but at my naked self. He sat in a chair beside the bed and pulled a contraption closer towards him. He then shook a bottle and squirted freezing cold gel onto my belly. Agghh...I recognised this. Shit, did they think I was pregnant? I knew I was a bit porky but that's just mean. He then soaked my legs in gel. I looked down and cringed, this poor boy, I wore a thong that was brandished with a delicate leopard print bow decoration. I blushed on behalf of this poor, poor young man.

The testing did continue the next morning. I had my boobs clamped, something I had never had the pleasure of experiencing before. I filled my urine sample but my stool pot remained unused. The next basement rollercoaster wheelchair venture was an internal. This unfortunately was another experience I was familiar with. Then back to the comfort of my little room where more blood was taken.

13

The Waggling Pipework

Lunch time arrived. I was becoming more comfortable with eating the combination of unusually coloured and unrecognisable food. Guess what – I hadn't researched Russian cuisine either. I certainly hadn't lost my appetite. Shortly after polishing off my lunch, a beautiful nurse came to transfer me to a bigger room. She, along with a porter, moved my bags, coat and everything over to this luxurious room, just off what I would discover to be the main lounge. While sat in my new room, I heard familiar voices outside my door laughing and joking. Most of the people I'd got to know a little from the forum were sat in the communal area. I left my room and went over to them, plonked myself down on the sofa and eagerly joined in with a very relaxed and easy conversation. A lot of the talk revolved around each person's journey so far, which very helpfully, served as stepping stones for us newbies. My smile changed quickly to a silent gasp, as a patient, a week further down the line, was wheeled into the lounge.

Two tubes protruded out of the side of this poor woman's neck. Every time she moved these antennae wiggled. It was like something out of a horror film. One of my fellow bucket wielders noticing my reaction smiled "you'll have those soon."

Oh my, maybe I should've looked into what the hell I was doing.

"They don't hurt, in fact I hardly notice them," said the antenna lady in a broad Dutch accent, as her neck tubing swung from side to side.

Every time she spoke I found myself distracted by her waggling pipework but then I was drawn back into the general vibe in the room. Our multicultural, uber-positive clan laughed and joked throughout the evening, anyone would have thought we were on holiday hearing us. We only stopped briefly for food, to have bloods taken or catheter bags emptied.

My next milestone was the head shave. Considering it was now about to become a reality, I stroked my curls to remind myself of what they felt like. Many of the MS fighters had shaved heads. The penny had dropped; it was all going to be coming off anyway once I had the poisonous chemicals pumped into me. I had no idea how the chemo was going to be introduced into my poor ignorant body, deciding instead to remain oblivious to what was going to happen and remove it regardless. After all, they do say ignorance is bliss.

Taking a deep breath, I put my tinted glasses back on. The amount I had spent over the years on conditioner was insane. I was going to save a fortune and imagine how quick I would be in the morning. Ooh and best of all - no more blocked drains. I had spent many cumulative hours on my knees twirling a cotton bud to extract hair from the clogged up plug hole of the bath. The regular hair plug removal system resembled twisting spaghetti onto a fork. My hair was so thick I had to brush it in the shower with conditioner on. I wouldn't have to do that again for a while at least. Maybe never again if my hair came back straight. I had a sinking feeling, I did love my easy up curls. I touched them again and reassured myself I would get through this.

I had been given many gorgeous head scarves

by the red-haired miracle and a client. The "you can do this" lady from the meeting and I had become good friends. She had met me in a car park with raffle prizes, fundraising buckets and mountains of enthusiasm and encouragement. Before I had set off for Moscow, we had met for breakfast before going for my wig fitting. That day would turn out to be one of the funniest of my life. She came to collect me with her hair looking gorgeous - straight out of a salon gorgeous. This was in fact a well-coiffured wig but you would never have known. Both of us, with sticks in hand, tottered off to the unbelievably talented wig maker. On a previous visit, he had studied my hair and ordered me a hair piece that was similar in texture and then dyed, highlighted, low lighted and curled the hair to look exactly like my natural locks.

She sat with me as he carefully fitted it. He showed me how to use tape to attach it to my scalp whilst I had hair, then how to glue it securely when I was bald. This information flew over my head at the time. The wig looked amazing and very authentic. The two of us left the hairdressers with our wigs on and sticks in hands. My fellow toddler suddenly grabbed my arm and we both went crashing to the floor in a heap. We burst out laughing through her giggly apologies as our sticks went flying in opposite directions. I managed to get myself upright and turned to her to witness two bulky looking builders lifting her to her feet. As they walked away, I just smiled, thinking "I should've stayed down." The laughter continued through breakfast and was heightened when she fell off her chair in the café. Humour is one of the best tools against any disease - MS definitely.

Breakfast with friends is one of my favourite pastimes. One of the three fundraising party trio (who would unknowingly become key to my recovery later) and I went to a quaint café out in the countryside for a bit of quality time together before I left the country. She helped me up the step and found us a table close by, then went off to order. We drank tea, ate scrummy food and chatted like there was no tomorrow. She asked how nervous I was.

"Just the hair thing," I admitted as I went to run my fingers through my mass of curls.

This seemed the appropriate response but I only managed about two centimetres through my locks before my fingers were greeted with a knot. A nail snagged on one of my curls, "ow."

"Right, lets sort it" she said beaming. "It's only a couple of months before you go, lets sort it," and with that she dragged me to a nearby hairdresser.

"What?" Surely she wasn't expecting me to cut my hair already.

No space, oh well clearly not meant to be.

"I'll ask our sister salon if they've a space, it's only a two-minute drive," said the salon receptionist (who looked like she just stepped out of a salon ironically).

Turns out they had a space. We rocked up and within seconds I was sat nervously in the chair, my loose hair flowing halfway down my back. The scissors came out to shouts of "shorter," and "you look beautiful." If encouragement and flattery could make this any easier, I was with the perfect companion. Within an hour I left about a stone lighter, where were scales when you needed them? I was a tad poorer but with confidence in my short 'fro.

I had a teeny bag containing my severed mane and a new hair product. What can I say - the hairdresser was so sympathetic and lovely she deserved the commission. I had planned to donate my hair to a charity that makes wigs for kids. I needed all the karma points I could get - I was off to Russia for medical treatment.

It was now the day of the shave. I was currently

sporting ear length curls. A very attractive dark haired, blue eyed nurse beckoned me. I did again wonder if Russian women were all naturally beautiful or if they only hired stunning nurses. They worked long shifts so surely they couldn't have time to prepare their gorgeous selves daily (unless they were all on speed.) I entered the clinical white room where there was a chair placed in the middle of the floor. She whipped out the electric clippers as if she were John Wayne pulling out his gun. A few smooth waves of her hand and I was de-haired. If only waxing was this pain free and quick.

I felt that I had now truly joined my equally bald comrades in the lounge. I intermittently wore headscarves but my head got so hot. How I survived with a thick lion's mane I have no idea. I didn't feel out of place as we were baldies together. My shaved look was actually very different to having a fully bald head, as I found out after chemo.

I had passed all the tests with flying colours, in fact, not that I like to boast but had excelled. My blood pressure was naturally low so the stress of the treatment had brought it to a normal level. My sinuses, heart, lungs and kidneys were all in great condition. Wow, maybe the University diet of Bacardi with noodles wasn't so bad after all.

I'm sure they made all the difference by soaking up the toxins. The only discovery by the clinic was the presence of 'squirls' situated in my lady parts. I nodded presuming they were talking about my coil. It was only back in England, when my physio pulled out my file and an ultrasound scan fell out, did I discover the true nature of the 'squirls.'

Looking at the scan on the floor I gasped "what on earth."

"It's your uterus," my physio said "you've got endometriosis."

Thank goodness for that. I didn't want any more kids.

Endometriosis is a condition which looks like webbing, it is very painful and can cause fertility issues. I had managed to get pregnant three times so perhaps my webbing was more of a hammock for my two. The third baby just wasn't ready for the world. I always had mild back pains during my cycle but excruciating was not an adjective I would use.

I sat upright in my adjustable hospital bed covered in crisp white cotton sheets that were laundered daily, pillows were fluffed to perfection. Early each morning a nurse would come and take my blood pressure and my temperature. This would be done regularly in between the frequent four times daily feeds. We also were left biscuits and baby food to snack on - no joke! My body was going to be pumped with steroids so I would almost be clawing at the door for food in the days to follow.

It was about 2am when I woke and my stomach growled. I had drunk copious amounts of tea, eaten four large meals, plus bread, accompanying biscuits and pudding the previous day. I climbed out of bed and was too ravenous to waste time adjusting the bed. I rifled through the wrappers on my bedside cabinet and the remnants of my pre-sleep biscuits. I looked in my snack drawer which was empty, how? It was full the day before. I needed food. I walked as fast as I could, dragging the drip stand across the room to the fridge. As the door opened I was greeted with a heavenly glowing light. The sum total contents were a protein shake and two jars of baby food. I was like an addict, twisting the cap off of the protein shake and downing it in seconds. It seemed reminiscent of chugging snake bite, not big or clever may I add. I then ripped the tin lids off the baby food and threw them roughly towards the direction of the bin, whilst grabbing a used teaspoon. I scoffed those jars of pureed baby food as if I had not eaten for months. It had been a couple of hours - madness!

The food presented to me so far had been largely unrecognisable. Not only was it hospital food but it was carefully measured, nutritionally calculated, Russian hospital food. Some meals were not the most desirable and I was grateful for the condiment warning. It only took a couple of days telling myself "this food is designed to keep me well," before I acclimatised and the seasonings weren't necessary and were cast aside like the wrappers of continual snacks I'd ravaged. The exception to the colourful calorie condensed foods were baked apples and large chunks of soft beef. It was so soft I did wonder if it had been lovingly pummelled by the hands of the stunning nurses during their short time away from the hospital.

The tubes placed into my neck looked gruesome and they were inserted in two stages. Again, I must admit ignorance to the procedure. I lay on my side as two nurses with scalpels, the tubes and I don't even know what else, stood at the side of my bed. I closed my eyes. I was not remotely phased by injections but scalpels to my neck was not something I wanted to watch. A bit like when I first had to jab myself. A bit of tugging later and I had tubes protruding out the side of my neck. There was no pain, so anaesthesia was clearly doing its part. At first I avoided looking in the mirror remembering the shock of seeing the 'antennae lady' and my introduction to 'neck wagglers.' I soon realised that injecting substances into your neck is the fastest and easiest access route. These would be my first set of 'wagglers' and is how my stem cells would be harvested.

Now, as number 9 will confirm, I can make anything a competition. The creator of our online July fighters group had the required number of stem cells harvested within about five hours. I joked with him and his gorgeous wife that my only aim was to beat his time. I haven't stated the fact that you need so many million in relation to your body size. Although I was growing a food belly I am only five foot 1 and a smidge if you recall. His six foot plus towered over me and so would surely need more stemmies. More stem cells would surely have equated to a longer harvest time. Turns out however, my theory was flawed.

I'd been accompanied twenty-four hours a day by drip stands containing bags of goop, which helped to increase stem cell production, protect my liver and kidneys and provide the obligatory pain killers. Chemo was going to be introduced later, after my stemmies had been harvested. That word "harvested" always makes me want to throw up a little bit and reminds me of the dystopian thriller film 'Soylent Green.' It is however, the correct term to use. The drips themselves didn't bother me as steroid infusions and Tysabri every month for the last six years had hardened me to those tubes.

I got used to the beeps going off in almost a chorus sound as the machines emptied different bags of gloop into my blood stream. My precious bag of baby stemmies were taken away and were spun to separate the naughty MS infected stem cells from the unaffected fresh ones. I never remember if the evil stemmies are the fatties or the nasty scrawny ones. Either way, the bad ones are banished, hopefully into a humiliating pot of freezing cold painful stabby needles. The warrior cells are frozen, in a calm heavenly womb like state I imagine, until their reintroduction later.

14

The Soft Russian Lullaby

The combinations of food continued to be welcomed by my ever ravenous, steroid filled self. Apparently most people lose weight during chemo. I however, managed to develop the most perfectly formed Buddha belly. I guess leaving my hair and waistline along with MS in Russia isn't such a bad deal though.

My tubes were removed and new ones put in their place. Rumour has it, I had tubes in both my heart and my spine? My ignorant state continued to remain a grace but still keeping me as hard-core as She-ra. I preferred it that way.

The food portions increased and I was told to eat more. Eat more – when do you ever hear those words! I started having sugar in my tea, a habit I'd managed to kick years ago, in an attempt to bump up my calorific consumption. Chemo time wasn't far off for me at this stage. I was put into isolation, which basically meant staying in my room with no visitors. My room was cleaned so regularly I'm surprised there was still any flooring or paint on the walls. Even the outside of my door was cleaned in case it was opened by a non-gowned person. I could understand one possibly gaining OCD after this experience.

Four days of the dreaded chemo begins.

I had contact with the rest of my little team while in isolation via our online group chat. This proved to be a very welcome lifeline.

I had a huge craving for bananas, something I'd mentioned to the group. The next day one of the nurses knocked on my door, with bananas in her hand. I have never been so overjoyed to see the yellow fruit in my life! A new arrival had read my plea in our chat box and picked some up for me as he arrived for testing. It was like that. Bonds were made with people you hadn't even met as we were all going through this unknown experience together.

The hippy scientist doctor came to see me every morning and every evening before he left to check my blood pressure. I don't think he ever actually looked at the results but soon realised he was just checking my well-being, as I was one of the few people there without a companion. This was clearly one of those jobs you do out of love not for the money. I expect his wages were relatively high in the Russian economy but I'm certain they wouldn't reflect the hours, dedication and patient care that he gave.

One of the nurses became my Russian mother figure and another nurse my Russian best friend. When my clothes were taken away and my sweet scented toiletries removed, these were the ladies that showed me which bottles of vodka to use for my body, which for my face, my nether regions and which was a substitute for a toothpaste. Different strengths of vodka and disposable soft netting cloths would replace my toothbrush, shower gel and other daily items. In isolation I learnt how to move rapidly to the loo with a drip stand in tow. At one point I must have had eight bags of gloop being dripped into me. The good doctor, AKA hippy scientist, spoke to me during one of the morning blood pressure checks and tried to persuade me to have a catheter fitted, something that I'd always associated with incontinence. I refused - I was proudly still dodging this common MS symptom. I was not about to give up this important autonomy. That night however, I tripped over my feet rushing to the toilet and hit the wall with the IV line from the drip still attached. The next day the doctor came and asked me again more persuasively this time. The fall had been distressing so I backed down and had the catheter fitted. It didn't hurt to have it put in but seeing this clear bag fill, without me realising it was surreal. The nurses came in regularly throughout the day and night to empty the bag into small jugs. They moved swiftly in the shadows carrying out this matter of fact task, allowing me to keep my dignity and claim ignorance of me having relented.

A few days after having it fitted, I awoke one night in the early hours to an excruciating pain from inside of me. The specialist nurse was called in and decided it would be for the best to have the catheter removed. I'm not sure what had happened but it wasn't comfortable. One of my regular and familiar nurses came to me and discreetly offered me a grown up nappy. The knowledge of their use I swore would remain in Russia with my waistline, hair and MS. I do however, want to be honest and open, even in my shame, as I put pen to paper.

Dignity is hugely stolen by MS. Taking that, to me, is more hurtful than any leg pains in the cold, the trembling and other after-effects of the regular injections. Even the years of regular self-harm with injections to slow down the evil monster pales in comparison. If I had to be introduced to nappies in my thirties this would to me, be an acceptable time and place. My multi-national team of "fuck it bucket" carriers would be going through their own challenges. These people held a bond with me that no one else will ever understand. They became, as the good doctor had said, my stem cell family.

Chemotherapy ends – 2 days to go before the transplant.

A huge worry before I embarked on this madness was leaving my precious children but I have never spoken to them as much as I did in this period. We talked several times a day and I became much closer to my teenage son. I just had to ensure my antennae were not showing and I wore a head scarf. The little lady would read me stories and included me (via the tablet) in her regular doll's birthday parties. The dolls had lots of birthdays.

Two days of the same routine followed, eager-ly in anticipation of the new stem cells and all the improvements they would bring.

The day of my stem cell birthday arrived. A rebirth with the introduction of my new clean stemmies to my newly MS free body. The good doctor entered the room with a team of nurses and a huge monitor. They attached various patches to me, which immediately showed my fast paced heart rate. All my checks were done then a typically beautiful nurse held aloft a medium sized bag of blood as she came into the room. "My dear, your stem cells."

One of my bucket holders' husbands filmed the whole thing for me. I'm glad because it's not ever going to happen again and it's a pretty cool experience. Literally. As my stem cells were introduced I shook as I felt the cold entering my system.

"Can you feel pressure on your chest?" asked the Doctor.

"It's so cold," I replied, my heart racing. I was short of breath.

"We will wait for a minute, are you okay?" the doctor asked as he looked at the monitor.

I felt scared now and so cold. I didn't know what my body was doing. I gritted my teeth.

"My dear, I will add warmth and then more stem cells."

The doctor held my hand. He was passed a syringe and then introduced the contents into one of my antennae. A few moments passed then he continued with the stemmies.

"Are you okay? Are you breathing okay? Any pain? Do you feel the pressure on your chest lessening?"

I forced a smile "I'm so cold."

I'd had a panic attack half way through. Due to an extreme lack of research, I hadn't expected the stem cells to be ice cold. In this and only this instance, ignorance was not bliss. Knowledge would have been power by preparing me for this strange experience.

Following the transplant, I would be in isolation for a further seven days. Firstly though, I had my stem cell party to attend. I had already attended two of these highly emotional celebrations. I went to the lounge and joined other patients, carers and nurses. We had yet more biscuits and cake.

As I had seen him do previously, the good doctor gave a powerful speech but this one was about me. He went onto say that although it had been testing, my positivity had kept me strong and we got through it together. Everyone clapped and cheered. Then the huge fire hydrant style thing was brought into the room. This was in fact liquid nitrogen that had kept the stem cells safe before transplant.

The good doctor and I ceremoniously tipped

out some of the liquid which evaporated quickly in a cold mist. Many claps and cheers of happy birthday brought a huge smile to my face, on this very first stem cell birthday and with it, an end to the progression of the MS monster and all the shit it had brought with it.

So many people had suggested I binge watched various series in my 'time out.' I tried but they bored me. I've never been a TV fan and prefer to take part in board games or enjoy a cuppa and a natter like a truly English girl. Board games are somewhat difficult solo and the card game 'Patience' gets boring after the first failed attempt. The majority of my time I spent listening to guided meditations, admittedly most were interrupted for new drips to be fitted into my neck, check my blood pressure, temperature or to feed me. I always remembered what the good doctor had said to me, "fifty percent science, fifty percent you. Meditate, do yoga and think good thoughts."

I was only sleeping about five hours a day so I managed to catch up with the kids, friends, and family. Luckily the people were in different time zones, so my 3am natter would be a reasonable time for one or the other. I did lots of focused breathing and relaxation techniques, things I'd been teaching for years so it was second nature to me. I recapped on a lot of my studies - things like massage, anatomy, essential oils and manifestation (visualising and focusing on something until it appears in your realm).

There were however, dark times when my rose-tinted glasses had slipped.

A family member with good intent had sent a link to a song that reminded me of the little lady and the tears came flooding out. I had to remind myself I was doing this for them and I think the release did me good.

The next was waking up one night with pains so severe I actually asked for pain killers. After a day of being violently sick, it became apparent that I have an intolerance to Opioids. No Tramadol or Codeine for me then. To be fair, it was probably my holistic inner self telling me to deal with the pain and breathe through the pain. I had something injected into my neck instead.

But possibly the worst of all happened shortly after chemo ended.

I had woken in the night and looked at my hands. They were covered in hair, as was my pillow, face arms and sheets. I knew it was going to happen but the knowing still hadn't prepared me for this. The silent tears came flowing, but my fluffy cat was in

England.

I pressed the buzzer on the wall. I'd been told off for not asking for help enough so now seemed appropriate, as there was no cat to comfort me. My heart throbbed, my bottom lip shook, my breath was shallow and the lump in my throat grew. Now was the time to buzz. A nurse arrived in seconds, took one look at me and instinctively went into the bathroom and returned with some damp cloths. She wiped my face, arms, helped me out of bed and then changed my sheets. She gently wiped over my head and popped on a hair net before helping me back into bed, nodding knowingly before leaving. Something so simple but at that moment, I had felt like a small vulnerable child and her caring presence was needed to fix what I couldn't myself.

The very next day I'd found my rose-tinted glasses. Sporting my blue hairnet, I went to the bathroom and rubbed at my top lip. Chemo would be replacing my regular waxing sessions. The hair on my top lip was minimal. I had been waxed before leaving for Russia, I'd wanted to look good for seeing clients, friends and family at the many fundraisers but nonetheless I rubbed at my lip, then my chin, armpits and legs. I was going to make the most of this unusual phenomenon and between you and me, my bikini had never looked so fabulous.

I have used hair removal creams, epilators, waxing, threading, and sugaring but none with such great effect. I was quite sickly though, so chemo is probably a bit too far for a stylish bikini line, if I'm honest.

Once my head hair had all come out I readily embraced the bald look, mainly driven however because I was always so hot. I had fluffy pyjamas ready for frosty Russia. It was July, and it turns out, hot in Moscow. Fortunately, they provided all patients with white cotton karate style PJ's, the comfiest clothes I will ever wear.

My time in Russia was coming to an end. The motherly nurse came in as she had done many times before. She had such a soft kind face. She signalled for me to lay down so that she could remove the neck tubes. On the white trolley beside me, were neatly arranged swabs and various medical tools. As I lay there on my side I started thinking about all of the treatment I'd had. All those weird and wonderful tests I hadn't even known existed. They were just to make sure my body was strong enough to handle the high dose of chemo. The dosage is much higher than is given for cancer as the entire immune system needs to be wiped, leaving just enough to keep you alive. The room had been cleaned so frequently and I hadn't even been allowed a toothbrush just in case I'd cut my mouth. This treatment had seemed pretty powerful. I was so glad I hadn't done much research as I probably would have backed out. I remember reassuring family and friends that I was going to be fine and that this was the best treatment. In hindsight I was just reassuring myself as I covered my ears and put my tinted glasses on. This was really scary stuff in an unfamiliar country, miles away from my family. The tears fell fast onto my pillow.

As I did so, the nurse drew closer to me, and just as I would imagine a Fairy Godmother to do, began to sing softly. As she sang what sounded like a Russian lullaby, she gently wiped away each tear. My pillow was damp from all of my tears of suppressed fear and relief that had come flooding out. She gently put her hand to the side of my face, moved away, then turned and nodded with a soft smile as she left the room. Just a few minutes later she returned. Sliding one arm under me, she pulled me up close as if to hug me and sat me upright. She then said something in Russian giving me that very familiar warm smile and left the room.

I was told off by the good doctor for stretching (now was not the time for yoga), being out of bed and unbelievably…not eating enough. How was that even possible? My immune system was still young and it needed nursing. I had protein shakes introduced to my diet alongside the biscuits and baby food. My body was getting stronger. By day 8 of isolation, I was given the go ahead to leave the room. Eight days was a pretty short burst for a new immune system to kick in. I believe it's usually longer. The blood tests however don't lie.

Preparing myself to join some of the others again, I stood up and walked towards the door. I heard a cough on the other side and swiftly retreated back to my bed, scurrying back like a little animal. I really didn't need to sit in the lounge. We could all talk on-line. I had the tablet for films and was happy listening to Audible books about reflexology, well-being and taking over the world with petals type hippy things.

I'd wait a few more days before leaving my safe haven, just to be sure. I hadn't come this far to only come this far. The next morning the good doctor came. He didn't even pretend to take my blood pressure.

"You can leave your room," he instructed.

I frowned.

"Your new immune system is strong enough now."

I was nervous. What if someone sneezed? He coaxed me out of the room. I took less than five steps to the sofa in the communal lounge. Three days later I was told that I was allowed to go outside in the hospital courtyard but that seemed excessive to me. The lounge was adventurous and nerve wracking enough for this month. Besides, I needed a lot of meditating to prepare myself to deal with the outside world and the dirty people who don't use vodka to wash. I had been anxious about going into the lounge and managed to side step venturing into the germ fest outside. I had to brace myself shortly for an airport full of strangers to embark on my journey home. The good doctor reassured me that with a mask and hand sanitiser I would be fine as my immune system was strong. He wouldn't let me go if it wasn't.

The Yorkshire man was heading to Russia to collect me and get me home safely. I was to remain in isolation once I got home, until my immune system was strong enough to handle the outside world. My young mum, number 9 and another friend had got together and gutted and cleaned my new downstairs bedroom, wet-room and kitchen.

I would need to wear masks if I saw anyone and remain in that portion of the house so it could be regularly cleaned. We could not afford to jeopardise my new MS free body.

15

The Blue Footed Booby

My time in Russia had come to an end. I had fallen in love with the city, its people and swore to return – albeit under different circumstances. I couldn't believe I had been here over a month. I was missing the kids and my home but my goodness was I scared. I had lived in this protected cocoon of people and an environment that made sure I was safe. I was amongst people who knew the treatment. I'd be leaving those who didn't blink an eyelid at the shameful lows but who also celebrated the huge emotional highs of a stem cell rebirth.

As I waved goodbye to the daunting uncertainty that MS brings, I just had to head home to try and soften the damage caused before I found Russia. I wasn't allowed to take the pyjamas, but my remaining vodka body wash and towelling cloths were packed in my suitcase like souvenirs from the trip. The many full condiments, I left in the lounge for new patients (just in case they did actually taste their food).

The Yorkshire man arrived. He squeezed my hand "I'm proud of you," and took my cases.

This was a huge step – back out into the outside world. I put on my headscarf, face mask and rose-tinted glasses. I waved goodbye to my Stemmie brothers and sisters and blew germ free kisses to the nurses. I had a long journey ahead to gain my strength and rewire my brain. To begin with I would be back in isolation for three months. Perhaps I could watch a series? Nah, I'll just meditate for now.

As the chauffeur wheeled me to the car I felt excited but apprehensive. The happy doctor and the team knew what they were doing. They knew what I should be eating and drinking and they knew what would ease my pain. I was heading back to my babies but what did I need to avoid? I had become accustomed to the flawless support, so stepping out I didn't feel like a powerful fighter, I was petrified. Taking those first tentative steps into the ward's lounge was one thing but into an airport of dirty, un-sanitised, unmasked humans was daunting.

As to be expected, the check-in went smoothly. I'm not sure whether it was the stern Russian decorum or my unusual attire that kept people at a safe distance. The sight of me in a surgical mask would have made anyone apprehensive. Whatever the reason, my nervous self was grateful. I was wheeled right up to the departure lounge sporting my headscarf, face mask and gloves. I was armed with sanitiser, antibacterial wipes and was under strict instruction not to eat anything that wasn't straight out of a packet. When it comes to food I'm not the most hygienic person I'll admit, extending the five second pick up rule of any dropped food to a minute or two if it's the last remaining food item (or particularly tasty) but I hadn't lost all my hair, left my babies for a month and been turned into something akin to a Dalek for nothing. Packet food only, no fresh fruit or vegetables (apparently these carry the most germies). No milk or fish, plus everything had to be super cooked and then zapped again. What was I meant to eat? I had no beautiful nurses to pummel beef in-between shifts. My young mum and the Yorkshire man were to be given my very precious new-born reins.

Standing to greet the passengers at the entrance of the plane was the classic blend of a beautiful woman and a perfectly made-up airhostess in a perfectly pressed smart uniform. I tottered onto the plane, handed my walking stick over to the Yorkshireman and prepared myself for the first step of a very long aisle of seats. From past experience, I would have to move in a monkey bar fashion, pushing off head-rests to keep me upright. Reassuring myself that the plane would have been thoroughly cleaned before each flight, my gloves would protect me from the germs nestled on the seats and surroundings. I just had to remember not to touch my face. My body was a brand-new golden temple.

I was amongst the first passengers to board so it was a good time to move through the cabin to find my seat. Less germies, for now, until the dirty passengers with their filthy kids boarded. I took a short, shallow breath as a deep one might suck in particles of dirt through any gaps in my mask. This was a surgical mask so it was highly unlikely but best not to risk it. The hostess beckoned me to a seat only a couple of steps away. This was business class, there must've been a mistake. Then I saw the Yorkshire man beaming. "We've been bumped up."

I'd never seen seats on an aeroplane like this

before. We had a mini pod each with loads of space, a swanky looking TV screen, a table, plus a welcome pack with a blanket, pillows, eye-mask and a branded toiletries bag. Wow, my own little cocoon for the journey back home.

"Not bad hey," said the Yorkshire man from his adjoining pod.

"Maybe it was worth the chemo," I said grinning.

The take-off seemed smoother than any I'd experienced before but I suspected that was partly down to my super luxurious business pod padding out any discomfort.

Once we were safely in the air, the hostess came and handed out menus that looked like they belonged to a Michelin star restaurant. Were we really several thousand feet up in the air? Every dish on the four-course menu would have made my taste buds sing. Reluctantly, I handed back my menu and explained that I was only allowed to consume food that was served in individual packets. My inner child, throwing a strop, crossed her arms and out came the bottom lip. My taste buds shed a tear. She nodded and took the Yorkshire man's order. "What a waste," I thought to myself. The choice of Braised beef and coke when he could have had salmon with spiced black lentils and a whiskey? C'mon. The airhostess reappeared after just a couple of minutes with her arms full. She pulled my table out and placed on it several chocolate bars, packets of popcorn, peanuts and crisps and then told me she would open a juice and pour me the first glass. My taste bud tantrum stopped and I took off my gloves, sanitised my hands and wiped down all my individual packets.

I finished off my teenager's idea of a dream dinner and popped on a film - Bohemian Rhapsody. I'd heard good things about it and sat, tapping my feet as the tear inducing film played. Then, as if timed to include in a book, 'We Are the Champions' bellowed into my ears as the plane hit the runway. I took one of my individually packed travel tissues and wiped my tears before sanitising my hands, then put on my gloves in preparation for the dirty airport germs.

We waited until everyone else had left the cabin before we disembarked. I thanked the airhostess for her kindness and followed the Yorkshire man off the plane,

"Wait there," he said looking around for something before speaking to one of the cabin crew.

"Excuse me, I've asked for assistance, where's the chair please?" As she replied she pointed towards the tunnel.

I took in a shallow breath and started walking at a snail's pace. My assistance was at the end of the long, enclosed passage. Now, I have to say, the Russian hospitality put the English to shame. They couldn't have been more forthcoming with their support. I dragged my weary legs slowly, towards some very welcoming plastic seats at the end of the seemingly never-ending tunnel as the cabin staff flew past. It was the furthest I'd walked in over a month. The Yorkshire man wiped the seat down with anti-bacterial wipes before I sat, then rushed off to find the assistance we'd booked. He returned looking quite fraught.

"We have to wait, they're understaffed."

We'd picked a week when the airport staff were on strike. He then went on, rather animatedly, to tell me all about them. He had plenty of time for several sighs and told me that it had been up in the air whether or not our flights were going ahead. Phew.

My lack of watching TV and therefore ignorance of current affairs, clearly showed. It turns out the Yorkshire man had been selective in his reporting of the real world to protect the tints on my glasses. A porter finally arrived, seemingly a little reluctant he handed over the chair and hurried away. Next, we headed off to retrieve our luggage. The Yorkshire man stopped, then parked me up out of the way in a quiet area near a wall, before battling through the dirty, unmasked, sweaty, dishevelled passengers to get my two huge cases as well as his own. I'd been in Russia a month, so it seemed acceptable that my bags were bigger than me. Unfortunately, the sugary teas, biscuits and endless supply of food meant that I definitely weighed more than all my luggage combined.

I expect he was thankful for having the wheel-chair though. Pushing me, dragging my cases, lap-top bag, rucksack and handbag on his back, as well as his own case (laden with mainly my bits) was proving to be a struggle. He spotted and then homed in on an unsuspecting member of staff. A few polite, somewhat grovelling words later and the kind-hearted individual fetched a luggage trolley, then helped with taking the bags to the car park. I'm almost certain I heard him mutter about being overworked and maybe he should have gone on strike too as he scarpered off. The Yorkshire man wheeled me next to the luggage and rang the airport parking company to return my freshly washed and germ-free car.

My car pulled up and the Yorkshire man rushed over and handed him some money, then returned to get me. "No, bags first. No one will pinch me - I've eaten too much. Grab the bags."

He meticulously packed the cases into the car and then after wiping down all the surfaces, helped me into the passenger seat. This wasn't done in a remotely gracious fashion. My body was exhausted and so I reluctantly had to succumb to having help. It was the middle of summer, so once safely in the car away from the dirty people, I removed my gloves and head scarf but left the mask in place. The Yorkshire man drove us steadily and uneventfully back to my house. We pulled up and he helped me out of the car, straight through the now sterile house, to my new downstairs (for a while) bedroom. The room had been deep cleaned and was looking spotless. The bed had been made with brand new sheets, a brand new cover, on a brand new mattress. Hanging from the ceiling was a lampshade clearly decorated by my little lady. It had Mum written in big blue letters and hearts in different colours all beautifully drawn by her little self.

I squirted on some antibac gel and noticed several cleaning stations with masks, gloves, booties and even big gowns alongside the hand gel. They'd clearly been busy. There were no messy sides, everything was spotless and all unnecessary items had vanished. My very own pristine Russian hospital at home. I stepped into the bedroom and looked out of the huge sliding glass door overlooking my beautiful garden, but something had changed.

"A roofless veranda" I screeched. The Yorkshire man and his dad had built raised wooden decking right outside my bedroom. I was to be in isolation for around three months until my new immune system could handle the germs of the great un-masked. Incredible - I could stare out and it would feel like being outside and when strong enough, I would be able to do just that. The wooden veranda would be a lifeline – an almighty big stepping stone leading directly from my isolated bubble to facing the dangerous outside world. Until that next step it could be my viewing platform. A little too similar to the screens in zoos but what a glorious background of my herb garden. I felt so special. The Yorkshire man and his dad had spent a long time sawing, cutting and smoothing out the most perfect 'roofless veranda.'

The kids were still staying with my young mum and Patrick or their dad alternately. They would be coming a few days later after I'd gotten a little stronger.

Just as if it had been planned, two faces appeared in my garden smiling at me from the new viewing platform. Number 9 stood there with an enormous grin with her husband (and someone who I consider a good friend) standing proudly beside her. Both were in full Taekwondo whites - not dissimilar to my beloved hospital PJs. She was soon to be going for her black belt grading. This was amazing but I had still beaten her on the beep test I said to myself. I was so excited to see her.

"You look really well" she said through the glass pane.

"I'm bald" I replied removing my head scarf to reveal my smooth scalp.

"It suits you, you look hot," she beamed.

We spoke through the glass effortlessly although they did look cold. Maybe I could handle this non-isolated isolation.

Shortly after they'd gone, I turned to my welcoming new bed. Whilst climbing my short self onto my bed for first time, the Yorkshire man went quiet. I turned and saw a big grin on his face. "Nicely done."

I looked at him confused.

"That knee bent on its own. You didn't swing across or lift your leg by hand."

I'd not even thought about this before but apparently it had been a massive difference.

That night I curled up in my pristine new bed linen, new pillows and duvet. If I felt pain, I'd now have to take tablets instead of the far superior drugs that had been frequently syringed into my neck antennae. I wouldn't be in close contact with anyone for a while. The Yorkshire man kept his mask on and blue booties. These were just the same as they wore in the hospital or the food factories I'd worked in as a student. The sight of these on people's feet made me giggle childishly as they reminded me of the beautifully named blue footed booby - a real bird I promise - Google it!

It would be a while before my mum or the kids would come into the house. Unfortunately, despite our genetic links, they were still included in the germ ridden unmasked brigade but we still had the IPads and we knew we were in the same city. It was hard to be in the house without the kids but as I was in the designated "germ-free" section, it was far from normal living.

It became routine for the Yorkshire man to spray and wipe down every surface that I may have possibly come into contact with. This was my new normal. When my precious but germ ridden children were here they must also be blue-footed boobies. They would be doing visits rather than sleeping at home as I didn't have enough energy to walk far, let alone do the cooking, washing or referee the usual television related disputes.

Having a shower exhausted me. The red-haired miracle told me she just slept for months. Why was I so awake? It felt as if the general morning fatigue had lifted. The days grew long and despite having the huge window to stare out of and Netflix and Audible to hand, I missed human interactions.

One morning the Yorkshire man was out, possibly gone shopping or at work. I crept through the kitchen feeling like a naughty child who was meant to be tucked up in bed. I passed the bleached threshold of the kitchen and into the non-sterile corridor.

I felt something brush against my feet. There were no silent tears this time but the cat came to me anyway. How did it stand with cats? He wasn't a very good hunting cat so no dead animals but I knew he proudly licked his own bum. There would be no kisses and I'd wash my hands after.

"Hello, you" I said scruffling his fur. "I've missed you."

Just a few steps away was the lounge and my pride and joy - my four-foot fish tank.

16

FFFYFT

My dad had a huge fish tank which was about twenty-foot long. In hindsight, I was a little girl so it may actually have been a tad shorter. The "Hoover fish" spent most of its days sucking on the glass. Just looking at him resulted in me having fits of giggles. This may have sparked my passion for keeping fish. As a little girl, I also kept my own goldfish in a small plastic fishbowl with a small plastic plant. Then as a student I kept Sea Monkeys in a Strongbow glass I'd acquired. Finally, as a grown up, I progressed to a real fish tank.

I'd spent many days in garden centres, which usually came with the obligatory aquatic section.

I often gazed at the beautifully coloured fish on display in the tanks. It was soon to be my birthday and I'd decided I was going to buy my first proper tank. Fish tanks are quite understandably pricey. My Mum and Patrick offered to put some money towards the new tank for me. I was so excited. I had a wad of rolled notes secured with a hairband in my bag and was eager to get onto the fish tank ladder.

I bought a tank. I also bought lighting, heaters, stones, plants, ornaments, aqua safe, salts and the fish themselves. You can plainly see the pennies turning into pounds and the pounds turning into the wads of rolled notes in my bag. This outlay was in stark contrast to Sea Monkeys in a borrowed pint glass from my student days.

I spent days setting the tank up, allowing the water and chemicals to settle to bring my aquarium to the perfect(ish) levels. Then came my new Mollies and of course, sucker fish. Whenever I, the kids and their father were sat together, their eyes would all be set in the same direction. The direction of the all action, bright flashes on a screen of that which controls society - the television. I was the only one whose eyes were looking in another direction.

My tank mesmerised me. The colourful, fluttering tails of the male Guppies, bright and beautifully decorated to entice the females. The females content with their plain colours allowing the males to show off around them. Guppies are live bearers and every so often tiny little swimmers would appear. The Bakewell Tarts would comment on how I was "the breeder." The trick? Do nothing much. After the initial set up I occasionally changed the water. Never have I ever done a water test. Sometimes, the expert Dr Google was consulted. Advice was found such as adding frozen peas for unhappy, constipated fish, or swim bladder treatment for those that were wonky. On the rare tank changes, I would ask their dad to help. Just carrying a cuppa resulted in wet patches trailed across the floor, so bowls of dirty fish water would have ended as the floor resembling a pond. This could have been quite gross, even to one with a fairly liberal three-minute rule. This must have been an irritating chore, especially to someone who didn't have any remote interest in my little gilled friends.

I loved the idea of a tank in the wall. An entire wall of fish to admire - amazing. We had bought our house and he was often doing little projects. Maybe this was another man thing? The fire had been condemned and so we had it replaced. The other side of the chimney breast had been boarded up. Their dad had used a hammer to break through the boarding to reveal a recess.

"You can put your fish tank there."

It was a tiny space. I would need to get rid of my hoover fish and downsize to a much smaller tank. I was secretly devastated but as he pointed out, it's what I wanted. I was getting a tank in the wall, kind of. When their dad revealed the miserly recess I knew that I'd be giving up my huge tank. On a positive, this was gifted to a fabulous cousin of their dad's. I think it may now be the home for a snake. To sell would have caused my heart to break and the buyer's nose also, well, in my imagination anyway.

When their father ended the relationship and I'd managed to keep the house, I came to realise that I could hold the fort for my two little people and silent cat by myself. It turns out I was even stronger than I'd realised. I could do this and in fact I already was. This was now my house and my rules. I made the decisions and called the shots. One of the first things I did was to buy myself a four foot "fuck you" fish tank. This was the tank from which the albino sucker fish was now greeting me. That's the fish story.

I'd crept from within my sterile part of the house, down the corridor and towards the front room. Up until now, this had been a designated waiting area for anyone entering the house. They would proceed no further through without firstly being disinfected.

I stepped cautiously with one foot into the lounge. The other remained in the hallway. I'm pretty sure it doesn't count if only one half ventures into "no man's land." I stood in the doorway looking adoringly at my tank. The sucker fish had come to the side closest to me as if to welcome me back. I smiled before sneaking back slowly into my permitted area. It would be a while yet before I'd be cleaning those beauties solo.

I had attempted to watch TV on my faithful tablet but just found it an irritating waste of time so I returned to my faithful guided meditations and Audible. It became harder to be without the kids but if they came near me with their germs it might put me at risk and all the insanity of Russia would prove to be pointless. It was the hardest three weeks of the whole saga but the day came. I got dressed and put my sculpted wig in place. I heard the front door and knew my babies were just feet away. I listened to the Yorkshire man giving instructions about wearing hair nets, blue booties, sanitising to the elbow and of course, masking up. I waited on baited breath, then heard the excitement of my little lady "mummy!" as she came running over to the sanitised side. My best smile was hidden under my surgical mask, but the sparkle in my eyes and the excitement in my voice said it all. I held her so tight, only letting go to pull my son towards us. He towered over me but was still my fragile little premmie. All of this was for them, I was going to get stronger and stronger. My rose-tints were sparkling. My young mum followed behind the kids but was scared to get too close. I was stronger than she realised - she'd made me that way but I'm guessing in her eyes I was still her baby girl, just with less hair. They stayed for only a couple of hours but would return the next day. Apparently my body needed time to heal. My mind disagreed - I'd never been so awake.

I got myself organised and arranged the happy doctor's requested blood tests for at one, two and five months down the line. These would show my Lymphocyte levels, which although still low, were improving, strong little She-Ra cells for my new immune system.

In reality, it was extremely difficult getting past the all-knowing oracles; the GP receptionists, in order to arrange a home visit. Ultimately, it took me having to speak to a senior partner and explain that I had a weakened immune system before this request was approved. Eventually a nurse came with gloves but no mask. This wasn't a massive issue as I kept mine on 24/7 and no doubt the Yorkshire man would be stripping the bed later.

Physiotherapy was next on the list. I was still weak but I'd started to Google and contact various neurophysio's - mostly private and the NHS would only provide in house treatment but I really wasn't ready, or willing, to drive. As I looked for pointers, I spoke to one of my fundraising party trio friends - she was in the industry. I knew she lectured in cardio-physio but she must be able to point me in the direction of a neuro-physio. We nattered away about how "it's all a bit of a blur" and "feels like someone else's story." She told me how proud of me she was and to not do my usual run before I could walk.

"So," I said "do you know any neuro-physio's?"

She burst out laughing.

"Me. I'm a neuro-physio."

"I thought you lectured in cardio?"

She sounded excited "I lecture in cardio and my patients are neuro."

Sometimes what you're searching for is right in front of you. I initially arranged for two sessions a week. I was fortunate that so many people had helped to raise so much funding. Our sessions were short as I was weak but my progress was definite alongside my hair growth. It turns out I have a great head shape. As the days passed, I kept forgetting to put my headscarf on and the wig was so hot. At first my son freaked out and would shout "scarf, scarf," pointing at my head but then he must have got used to it or just gave up. On the unusual day I actually put the wig on, the little lady just said "it looks weird, take it off."

So, that was that. I was quite fond of my GI Jane do and rocked the bald look. As my hair began to grow, I thought back to all the crazy ideas of blond and straight or whether it would be red flowing hair. Turns out it was still dark. As for the "Chemo curls," this was just how it was before it thinned out whilst on Tysabri. Unfortunately, my leg, under arm, facial and bikini hair also invited themselves to the after party.

My motivational-haircut-prompting-physio (and friend) would come masked and gloved. She taught me how to adjust my posture and movement, starting with basic exercises that seemed so simple, but fuck me they were hard work. The effort and brain power it took to try and persuade my knee to bend was exhausting. I kept practising movements that toddlers do automatically. It was frustrating to struggle with what used to come so naturally.

I did have moments of anger. Why was my body not doing what it was told? I know I've probably drank too much and partied too hard but I did loads of exercise. I'd meditated, cut out gluten and dairy, been kind to people and was generally a good human being. Why was it so bloody hard to do what everyone took for granted? There are nasty people in this world. Why had karma decided I had to learn to walk so many times? What had I done wrong?

Silent tears escaped.

My gorgeous physio kept me moving forward both literally and emotionally. It was during these times of frustration that I needed her most. Stress plays a huge part in healing and this was about to become even more apparent.

I was resting in bed one afternoon, awake and preparing myself for the trauma of getting up. My phone started buzzing, it was the kid's dad "have you spoke to Liz recently?"

I'd spoken to my musketeer a couple of weeks ago, nothing major, just our usual nattering. Why was he asking?

"I've just read it on the news. I'm sorry."

The exact wording of the rest of the call escapes me, but just enough was said to start my mind spiralling and a sickening feeling clench my stomach.

This couldn't be right. I hung up and rang her number. I had three numbers for her. She was always losing or breaking her phones. No-one picked up. I left lots of frenzied messages, the standard content as I had done many times before.

"Monkey, its Kezia, ring me."

I frantically clicked on Facebook and looked for her profile. There was a friend request from her? What? I found her sister on my friends list and quickly typed away.

Hi it's Kezia, I can't get hold of Liz. Has she got another new phone?

I looked through all the messages that I'd sent her sister over the years, all with similar content. I can't get hold of your sister. Can you tell her to ring me?

This was just going to be like all the other times.

I got a reply about an hour later, can I ring you? I didn't want her to. She had never called before, just text me the number, why did she need to call?

No, I was too busy she'd have to call later.

Part of me already knew. I typed a standard polite reply as if on autopilot.

"Hi how are you doing? I'm plodding along, improving, but too slowly for my liking," then put my phone number. The phone rang, I plastered a huge smile on my face and took a deep breath and answered.

"Hi, I'm glad treatment went well, I've been watching your videos." Then she told me what I deep down already knew.

My disability is something that has, over the years been harder and harder to hide, but now it was there in your face. The wonky leg, bald head, mask and old lady stroller that the Yorkshire man had bought me, just until I was strong enough. This particular walker was a burnt orange colour so a bit funkier than the bog-standard metal ones.

Our third musketeer had a hidden disability. Her mind was poorly. I remembered back to my Uni days and that all of us were hiding something. An actor is the best job in the world to disguise who you really are, what you've faced and to mask your hidden demons.

The tears came crashing fast. I couldn't even

turn them into silent tears. I sobbed like a baby. I don't think I'd ever cried this hard, even when my own dad died. Mentally we're prepared and can rationalise if it were parents or anyone older but this was one of the musketeers. The three of us were going to grow old together. She'd taken me on a pub crawl, by taxi. We had so much to do together still. I had to show her I was going to beat MS. We were meant to be going on a proper pub crawl with me walking beside her. She wasn't allowed to leave me. She had been fighting with her mental health for years, her fight had been silent and harder than mine. She was fighting on every waking minute and possibly in her nightmares too. I miss her dearly and like so many who have lost someone, as cliché as it sounds, would give anything for just a few more minutes of their time.

A couple of days later, when I had the next physio session, I could hardly stand, let alone walk. The tears wouldn't stop and I just sobbed but reassuring as ever, it was pointed out that this was a prime example of the effects stress could have. We plodded on with the physio sessions. I'd improved over the last few weeks but now it seemed I'd taken several steps backwards. We kept at it and after several months, managed to get back to the stage I was at.

Slowly I continued to improve from there.

I meditate often, as my body responds to how clear my mind is. I think back to my happy, hippy Russian doctor and how he explained the importance of positivity and mental attitude. "You deal with what's in here (pointing to his head)." "Do yoga, meditate and I'll do the other fifty percent which is science."

So it's official, mental well-being and the physical body clearly go hand in hand.

My hair is growing fast - thicker and darker than before and wow, the Chemo curls are hard-core. I'd heard about these and my hair was always naturally super curly but these were next level spiral curls. My greys? Gone.

I am no longer a slave to a monthly infusion or injecting myself every other day. I don't worry about contracting a potentially fatal brain disease from the very drugs that were making me better. I've left my MS, my waistline and old haircut in Moscow. As a bonus, the grey hairs did not get past customs.

I'm not running, not yet anyway. I'm staying optimistic though but if I don't, let's be honest, you can see a better world when you take a leisurely stroll, peering through rose-tinted lenses.

Rose-Tinted

Connect with me

Email:

Kezia@rosetinted.me

Facebook:

https://www.facebook.com/rosetintedtales

Twitter:

https://twitter.com/RoseTintedMe

Instagram:

https://www.instagram.com/rosetintedme/